P9-DTF-733

Rationality and Compulsion

RENEWALS 458-4574

DATE DUE

WITHDRAWN
UTSA Libraries

International Perspectives in Philosophy and Psychiatry
Series editors

Bill (K.W.M.) Fulford
Katherine Morris
John Z Sadler
Giovanni Stanghellini

Volumes in the series:

Mind, Meaning, and Mental Disorder
Bolton and Hill

Postpsychiatry
Bracken and Thomas

Reconceiving Schizophrenia
Chung, Fulford, and Graham (ed.)

Nature and Narrative: An Introduction to the New Philosophy of Psychiatry
Fulford, Morris, Sadler, and Stanghellini

The Oxford Textbook of Philosophy and Psychiatry
Fulford, Thornton, and Graham

Dementia: Mind, Meaning, and the Person
Hughes, Louw, and Sabat

Body-Subjects and Disordered Minds
Matthews

The Metaphor of Mental Illness
Pickering

Trauma, Truth, and Reconciliation: Healing Damaged Relationships
Potter

The Philosophy of Psychiatry: A Companion
Radden

Values and Psychiatric Diagnosis
Sadler

Disembodied Spirits and Deanimated Bodies: The Psychopathology of Common Sense
Stanghellini

Forthcoming volumes in the series:

What is Mental Disorder?
Bolton

Empirical Ethics in Psychiatry
Widdershoven, Hope, van der Scheer, and McMillan

Rationality and Compulsion
Applying Action Theory to Psychiatry

Lennart Nordenfelt

Professor of Philosophy of Medicine and Health Care
at the Department of Health and Society
Linköping University
Linköping, Sweden

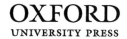

OXFORD
UNIVERSITY PRESS

OXFORD

UNIVERSITY PRESS

Great Clarendon Street, Oxford OX2 6DP

Oxford University Press is a department of the University of Oxford.
It furthers the University's objective of excellence in research, scholarship,
and education by publishing worldwide in

Oxford New York

Auckland Cape Town Dar es Salaam Hong Kong Karachi
Kuala Lumpur Madrid Melbourne Mexico City Nairobi
New Delhi Shanghai Taipei Toronto

With offices in

Argentina Austria Brazil Chile Czech Republic France Greece
Guatemala Hungary Italy Japan Poland Portugal Singapore
South Korea Switzerland Thailand Turkey Ukraine Vietnam

Oxford is a registered trade mark of Oxford University Press
in the UK and in certain other countries

Published in the United States
by Oxford University Press Inc., New York

© Oxford University Press, 2007

The moral rights of the author have been asserted
Database right Oxford University Press (maker)

First published 2007

All rights reserved. No part of this publication may be reproduced,
stored in a retrieval system, or transmitted, in any form or by any means,
without the prior permission in writing of Oxford University Press,
or as expressly permitted by law, or under terms agreed with the appropriate
reprographics rights organization. Enquiries concerning reproduction
outside the scope of the above should be sent to the Rights Department,
Oxford University Press, at the address above

You must not circulate this book in any other binding or cover
and you must impose this same condition on any acquirer

British Library Cataloguing in Publication Data

Data available

Library of Congress Cataloging-in-Publication Data

Nordenfelt, Lennart, 1945-
   Rationality and compulsion : applying action theory to psychiatry : an introduction
to the theory of action and its applicaitons to psychiatry / Lennart Nordenfelt.
      p. ; cm. -- (International perspectives in philosophy and psychiatry)
   Includes bibliographical references and index.
   ISBN 978-0-19-921485-3 (pbk.)
   1. Compulsive behavior--Psychological aspects. 2. Irrationalism (Philosophy) 3.
Delusions. I. title II. Series.
      [DNLM: 1. Compulsive Behavior--psychology. 2. Delusions--psychology. 3. Mental
Disorders--psychology. 4. Psychological Theory. 5. Rationalization. WM 176 N829r 2007]
RC533 .N63 2007
616.85'84--dc22   2006101658

Typeset by Cepha Imaging Pvt Ltd., Bangalore, India
Printed in Great Britain
on acid-free paper by
Biddles Ltd., King's Lynn

ISBN 978-0-19-921485-3 (Pbk.)

10 9 8 7 6 5 4 3 2 1

Library
University of Texas
at San Antonio

Contents

Preface

The systematic work on this book started during my sabbatical leave in Coventry, England, in 1998 and 1999. I then had the privilege of being a Visiting Professor at the sparkling Department of Philosophy at Warwick University, which for me, with its mixture of analytical and continental approaches to philosophy, was a great source of inspiration. I was given the best facilities for academic work, and for this I wish to express my gratitude to several people, including Mr. Greg Hunt who was then Head of Department, Mr. David Miller, Professor Michael Luntley, and, in particular, the head of the section for Philosophy and Mental Health, Professor K.W.M. (Bill) Fulford.

Since that time the project on action theory and mental illness has been interrupted many times by other engagements, among others a book project on animal health and welfare completed in 2006, but it has always been kept alive to some extent. The person who has all along in a gentle way reminded me about the topic is Bill Fulford, who is an admirable inspirer and supporter of scholars in the field of philosophy and mental health. Bill has several times joined the Scandinavian Group for the Philosophy of Mental Health at its annual meetings and he has continuously informed myself and others about developments in the area. He was also the person who told me about the OUP series on the philosophy of psychiatry.

During the final stage of the production of this book, I have been helped by a number of close colleagues in Sweden who have read the whole manuscript or parts of it. I wish, in particular, to mention Dr. Per-Anders Tengland and Mr. Erik Malmqvist. Let me also express my gratitude to some anonymous reviewers at OUP for their pertinent criticisms and remarks.

Since I have previously written extensively on action theory and the theory of health I have been able to use some arguments, and even a few complete passages, from works of mine that have been published earlier. With regard to action theory this holds for chapters 2 and 4. The main source for many of the distinctions there is my book: *Action, Ability and Health: Essays in the Philosophy of Action and Welfare* (2000) Kluwer: Dordrecht. My reasoning on the distinctions between competence and ability was first presented (1997) in 'On Ability, Opportunity, and Competence: An Inquiry into People's Possibility for Action'. In: G. Holmström-Hintikka and R. Tuomela (eds.) *Contemporary Action Theory. Vol. 1: Individual Action.* Synthese Library, Vol. 266, pp. 145–158.

I re-use parts of this material with kind permission of Springer Science and Business Media. With regard to the theory of health presented in Chapter 3, the main source is my *Health, Science and Ordinary Language* (2001) published by Rodopi, Amsterdam.

Now that I am making the final preparation of the manuscript for the publisher I am again using the opportunity of having a sabbatical year, this time in Sweden at the Swedish Collegium for Advanced Study in the Social Sciences (SCAS) at Uppsala University. I wish to extend my thanks to the Board of the Collegium and its Principal, Professor Björn Wittrock, for providing me with this new opportunity for systematic research. As on several previous occasions, Mr. Malcolm Forbes has given me substantial help in putting my English into publishable condition.

Lennart Nordenfelt
Uppsala, October 2006

General introduction

This book has three basic purposes. First, it is an introduction to philosophical action theory. It presents the basic notions surrounding the concept of action and attempts to show their interrelationships. In this regard, the text draws upon the extensive literature on mind and action that has followed upon the writings of Ludwig Wittgenstein (1953) and Gilbert Ryle (1949). Second, the book offers a development (much beyond elementary analysis) of such crucial notions within action theory as are particularly relevant for my third purpose. Among these notions are the ones of ability, rationality, and compulsion. Third, the book presents an analysis of the concepts of health and, in particular, some aspects of mental disorder, this on the basis of certain insights from action theory.

The book is a result of two diverging interests of mine: one is my life-long interest in the rational explanation and determination of action, the other is my interest in the theory of health. The first interest has led me to the development of a comprehensive theory of action-explanation, where the agent's intentions and beliefs are the main ingredients. The second interest has led me to the development of a theory of health based on the notion of human ability.

In previous studies, I have only combined these theories in my characterization of the general theory of health and welfare. Although I have, for a long time, seen the relevance of action theory to the understanding of some aspects of mental disorder, I have only occasionally made use of concepts from action theory in a psychiatric context. (For example, see my analysis of crime and accountability (1992 and 2000).) This could be seen as surprising since, first, mental ill health is so tightly connected to deviant human action and, second, the defects constituting mental ill health are often assumed to lie in the person's reasoning and action deliberation.

For some time now I have felt prompted to use action theory in an analysis of the machinery of mental disorder, and in particular in an analysis of some of the specific mental disorders. I am extremely aware of the complexity of the field of mental disorder and mental illness and of the fact that there is no reasonable hope of finding any characterization or explanation of mental disorder and illness in its entirety. The main, but not the only, pathological feature that I will comment on in this work is *delusion*, a feature which is central in most variants of schizophrenia but which is common also in several other illnesses, such as mania and paranoia (or, as it is sometimes called, 'delusional disorder'). (For extensive discussion about this, see for instance Oltmanns and Maher 1988 and more recently Amador and Kronengold 2004.) Delusion, whatever its precise definition, involves some alleged defect in the subject's understanding of the world. It thus mainly concerns the cognitive part of the human mind, although, as is argued by Fulford (1989; 2004) and others (including Cutting 1999), not exclusively so. I intentionally use the term 'understanding' and not 'belief' in this preliminary characterization of delusion. A specific reason for this is that some contemporary theorists have disputed that all delusions are of the belief kind. Other notions for mental states such as understanding, experience, and attitude have instead been suggested, in order to cover the variety of states that are currently denoted as delusions.

The analysis that follows has two main parts. Part 1 deals with action theory and introduces the main action-theoretic concepts. It also develops a theory of explanation of actions and gives a substantial analysis of ability in relation to human actions. Here I mainly draw upon my previous work in the field (1995; 2000). The section on mental ability, however, is a novelty in this book. In Part 2, I attempt to use the conceptual tools developed in the action-theoretic part for a discussion of topics relevant to psychiatric theory. The emphasis in the analysis lies on the notions of irrationality and compulsion. These notions, in particular irrationality, are commonly cited in psychiatric textbooks and deserve a careful analysis. I draw heavily upon the action-theoretic concepts in the analysis of irrationality and discriminate between several interpretations of irrationality. I find that some of these interpretations, but by no means all of them, are relevant to psychiatry.

The notion of compulsion is, I find, more promising as a tool for characterizing the typical action-theoretic features of several mental disorders. Even more adequate as such a tool is the combination of compulsion and irrationality, in particular such irrationality as disables a person from realizing his or her vital goals. By using this expression, I open the door to my own general characterization of health that will guide some of my final conclusions in the essay. In order to set the stage for the psychiatric analysis, I will therefore first give a presentation of my theory of health. I will in the conclusion give some concrete illustrations of my general ideas as applied to central psychiatric diagnoses, such as paranoia, phobia, obsession, and psychopathy.

The audience to which I direct myself is primarily psychologists and psychiatrists with a particular interest in the theoretical characterization of mental disorder and its various species. This is why my action-theoretic introduction is in part quite basic. However, I also direct myself to colleagues among philosophers who take an interest in the concepts of irrationality, compulsion, and mental disorder. My frequent use of the practical syllogism in the analysis of phenomena of irrationality and compulsion is, I hope, helpful in making a number of crucial distinctions in the area. My own analysis of compulsion is different and hopefully more accurate than some major previous analyses.

The presentation has the following structure:

Chapter 1, *Elements of the Philosophy of Action*, contains a treatment of several central action-theoretic concepts. The concept of intention is introduced and its crucial place in the determination and identification of actions is discussed. I give a substantial account of the different ways in which an action can be described and of how various descriptions can be compatible with the idea of action identity. The fact that actions occur in complexes, i.e. that one action can generate another action performed by the same agent at the same time, is further analysed. I also initiate an analysis of the notion of rational action and its relation to norms. This is a topic to be much more deeply discussed in Part 2.

Chapter 2, *On the Possibilities for Action: Ability, Opportunity, and Competence*, introduces the basic concepts of ability, opportunity, and competence and gives an account of the variety of factors that are prerequisites for the performance of actions. This chapter draws on my earlier analyses in *Action, Ability and Health* (2000) as well as on my article in Holmström-Hintikka and Tuomela (1997). My aim here is to give a systematic account of the conditions for action as well as of the parallel conditions for failure of action. I introduce a crucial distinction between first- and second-order ability, which is central to my further analysis of health. I also attempt to distinguish the notion of ability from a similar but distinct notion of competence.

In Chapter 3, *Towards a Theory of Health and Illness*, I summarize my account of the notions of health and illness that has been presented at many places before, in most detail in my 1995 and 2001. The presentation of health follows here since it directly builds on the previously introduced concepts of ability, in particular the concept of second-order ability. The basic idea that will guide my analysis later on is that a person is completely healthy if, and only if, this person has the second-order ability to realize all his or her vital goals given a specified set of circumstances. In this chapter, I also include a preliminary analysis of the notion of mental ability.

In Chapter 4, *On the Understanding and Explanation of Actions*, I distinguish first between the understanding of an action, i.e. correctly identifying and classifying an action, and the explanation of an action, i.e. explaining why an action has been performed. The focus in the chapter lies on the intentional and rational explanation of action. I argue that most (if not all) species of action-explanation are variants of a basic form of intentional explanation. In order to explain this, I introduce the idea of a *practical syllogism* that will play a central part in the rest of the book.

Chapter 5, *Reasons for Action and Rationality*, provides a platform for understanding the notion(s) of a completely rational action. I deal at length with issues of rationality and differentiate between different kinds of rationality. I then make substantial use of the notion of a practical syllogism and introduce a new syllogism based on the notion of a want. I also attempt to demonstrate the nature of *rationalization* of action, which is the particular relation that reasons take to actions in a deliberative situation. I say that a certain set of wants and beliefs of an agent A can rationalize A's acting in a certain way.

Chapter 6, *On Defective Rationalization of Action*, is more focused on issues of direct relevance to psychiatry. The chapter contains accounts of several interpretations of irrational wants and beliefs, as well as an analysis of the notion of defective rationalization. In chapter 5, I have asked myself: What conditions should be fulfilled in a perfect deliberation? From there I have the possibility of discerning the manifold ways in which a deliberation can go wrong from the point of view of the ideal. All human beings often fall short of the ideal in some respect. Such shortcomings might, but need not, indicate the presence of a mental disorder.

Chapter 7, *Towards a Theory of Mental Disorder: The Place of Compulsion*, moves the discussion closer to psychiatric issues. So far I have commented on psychiatric interpretations only in a negative way. I have noted that many instances of alleged irrationality (in the various senses) exist that do not warrant psychiatric interpretations. Everybody has his or her large share of irrationality. Most of us entertain some incoherent beliefs, the incoherence of which we have normally not yet discovered. Almost all of us have some unjustified beliefs, and some of us can have an illogical want-structure. Mental disorder is the case, I argue, only when *a genuine and enduring disability* in rational thinking and acting occurs. Here I am referring to the kinds of rationality that are necessary conditions for realizing something important to the subject – in line with my general analysis of health. Often this limitation of rationality is due to some form of compulsion. The notion of compulsion, therefore, is subjected to a substantial analysis.

Chapter 8, *Towards a New Analysis of Compulsion*, develops the idea that the notion of compulsion that is relevant in psychiatry is one tied to subjective unavoidability. This notion in its turn is based on the idea of fixation of intentions and convictions (beliefs or other experiences). A person A is subjectively compelled to perform a certain action F if, and only if, A's intentions and convictions are fixated in the sense that A cannot, or is absolutely not prepared to, change them. The fixation may be due to the subject's own choice but in the case of mental disorder it is typical that at least one of the two types (intention or conviction) has been implanted without the agent's own making. In special cases of mental disorder, such as automatism, the fixation may be due to the unavailability of alternative intentions and/or convictions.

In Chapter 9, *Compulsion and Specific Mental Disorders*, I attempt to substantiate my claim about the crucial place of compulsion by considering a number of specific mental disorders. I have found that my analysis can be applied, for instance, to the phenomena of paranoia, pathological drives such as kleptomania and pyromania, obsessions, phobia, rigidity, and psychopathy. My conclusion is that compulsion in my general sense of the word is a central element in all these conditions.

Part 1

Prolegomena to Action Theory and the Theory of Health

Chapter 1

Elements of the philosophy of action

1.1 **Introduction**

There is an exciting shift of focus today in many of the health sciences from the area of diseases and impairments to the area of ability, health, and quality of life. The WHO has for a long time emphasized a positive notion of health, but this notion has had little impact in the ordinary teaching of medicine. However, the health promotion movement, symbolized by for instance the Declaration of Ottawa, as well as the Association of Healthy Hospitals, has called for a development of a positive concept of health. The change of focus is particularly evident within the rehabilitative and the paramedical sciences. Several contemporary works in movement science (a branch of physiotherapy) and occupational therapy are among the leading forces in this development.

One crucial step in the development was of course also the introduction of the *International Classification of Impairments, Disabilities and Handicaps (ICIDH)* (1980) and its successor the *International Classification of Functioning, Disability and Health (ICF)* (2001), which presented for the first time a nomenclature for consequences of diseases, not least such overall consequences as entailed the subject's restricted ability to cope with his or her life roles. Thus, the concept of handicap was formally introduced into the medical vocabulary.

This general interest has prompted a lot of theoretical and conceptual work. Various systems and hierarchies of concepts have been constructed and defined. There is often much ingenuity and much important observation behind these constructions. One can, however, also see examples of unnecessary complications and even confusions in some of them. (I have in mind the recent classification *ICF*. For a commentary, see Nordenfelt 2003.) It is sometimes striking that these systems have not been guided by insights gained in philosophical action theory, a subdiscipline of philosophy that has existed since the times of the Greek master philosophers. In particular, Aristotle made a great number of important observations about actions, mainly in his works *Physics*, *Metaphysics*, and *Nicomachean Ethics*. Several of these observations have been used and been developed by modern action theorists. See in particular the works of Kenny (1963; 1975), Moya (1990), and A.R. Mele (1997). A modern *locus classicus* is G.E.M. Anscombe's *Intention* (1963).

This text has two purposes. It is an attempt to introduce, and at the same time develop, the philosophical analysis of action and ability in general. At the same time, however, I wish to indicate in what way I find action theory to be fruitful for the construction of conceptual systems and theories in the health sciences in general and psychiatry in particular.

1.2 **Action theory and its complications**

The field of actions is fascinating. Actions form a category with which we are extremely well acquainted. Every day we perform a multitude of actions, from the easiest and most trivial ones, such as washing our hands and having breakfast, to more complex and durational ones, such as communicating with our colleagues and running a business. We perform some of these actions without reflecting on them, or even without being aware of them. Some of them are performed almost automatically. Others, normally the more complex ones, require a large amount of both physical and mental energy.

The category of actions is, as I said, well known. On the other hand, it has proved to be quite difficult to characterize. The reasons for this are multifarious. First, actions are abstract objects. We cannot observe them with our senses and pinpoint them in the way we can directly observe and pinpoint physical objects. Somebody may contest this and say that actions may not be physical objects, but are they not physical events? Can we not observe a person who walks or drives a car? Is there anything abstract about such an event?

My answer to this, which I will argue in detail below, is that we may be able to observe some components of actions, namely their physical movement parts, but there are several other components that we cannot observe.

Second, and constituting a corollary of the fact that actions are abstract objects, it is difficult to find criteria of identity for actions. Under what conditions can we say that one action is the same as another one? And under what conditions is it important to be able to say that actions are identical or different?

Third, a great variety of actions exist. We can wonder what are the common elements in entities as distinct as moving one's arm, waiting for a bus, hammering in a nail, thinking about one's dissertation, opening a bank account, marrying someone, and leading a government. What are the common and general things that can be said about these disparate episodes?

Fourth, the action-language is extremely rich. We can describe actions in many ways and all these ways seem to be true and adequate. We can say of a man who is handing over a book to some person that he is performing the action of reaching his hand out to him or her. At the same time, he is giving the person a book. Moreover, at the same time, he may be keeping a promise as well as showing his gratitude to this person. Here are at least four descriptions of the same action performed by one single agent. But are they just four descriptions? Are there also four actions performed? Are these four actions different or identical? Here is one of the deepest and most difficult questions in action theory.

Fifth, how are actions to be explained and understood? Do actions belong to the physical universe, to be causally explained in physical or more precisely neurophysiological terms? Or, do actions form part of the phenomenological world of human beings, where they are to be explained and understood in a humanistic context of norms, reasons, and intentions?

These are some of the basic questions that I will confront in this book. I shall answer them as impartially as I can. A few of my answers follow a main stream of thought. In certain cases, however, where I have done basic research of my own, the answers will be more original, though still, I hope, well argued.

1.3 The nature of actions: actions and intentions

The basic question in action theory is of course: What is an action? How do we distinguish between actions and other kinds of behaviour? Why is my going to the university an action, while my falling to the ground in a heavy storm is a non-action? The traditional, and intuitively very plausible, answer has been to say that the former is an action because it is purposeful and intentional whereas the latter is not. When I go to the university I intend to go to the university, but when I fall to the ground my falling does not normally issue from any intention of mine. Thus, actions presuppose agents who make plans for their lives and form intentions according to these plans. A piece of behaviour that issues from such intentions is a proper human action. Other kinds of behaviour, or other kinds of bodily movements in general, including the inner working of the human body, fall outside. Bodily movements are important ingredients in many, though not all, human actions, but they are never sufficient to constitute an action.

If an intention is such a crucial feature of action one must ask: What sort of thing is an intention? What is the feature that distinguishes a stone's slipping from the hand of a man and this man's dropping the same stone? The two events may look identical. A physical examination of the hand of the person as well as of the course followed by the stone may give the same results in the two cases. Still, one of the two episodes is an action, the other is another kind of event involving bodily motion.

An intention is a mental state of affairs. I will say that an intention is a variant of a will. Other variants of will are wants and desires. There is a close connection between all these. A want typically issues in an intention, but it need not. A man who wants to get some food in the closest grocery shop typically decides to go there. And when he decides, he forms the intention to go to the grocery store, an intention that will exist in his mind until the moment when he arrives at his destination. However, persons can hold wants which are so unrealistic that they will never act upon them; for instance, they may want to become Olympic medalists, but since they realize that this is an idle wish, they will never *decide* to act on such a want.

The important difference between a want and an intention thus is that an intention is closer to an action than a want is. When persons intend to act, they are not – subjectively – unrealistic about the action in question. They believe that they can act in the way they intend. This is a conceptual point. It is, I would say, a *contradictio in adiecto* to say that people can intend to travel to Mumbai without their believing that it is possible for them to go to Mumbai.

An intention is a kind of strong will. An intention is always acted upon (if it lasts to the time when it is supposed to issue in action). An attempt to act at time *t* always exists if an intention to act at *t* exists. The things that can prevent an intention from succeeding have to do with the actual capacity of the agent – the agent can be mistaken with regard to his or her capacity – and with the external situation. Something can prevent the agent from acting in the way intended; an obstacle may exist on the ground or some other person may physically prevent the agent from succeeding in the attempt to act.

But what more specifically is an intention, what kind of mental state is it? I take an intention to be a kind of propensity to act in a certain way. It is a propensity to act in such a way that a particular goal will be obtained. Or, to put it into more precise terms: if A has the intention to reach a goal G, then A is disposed to perform all those actions which A considers necessary for reaching G. This propensity will issue in the right action if A is capable of and unprevented from acting. (For a development of this analysis of intentions, see Nordenfelt 2000.)

So far, however, I have not made any distinction between human beings and machines. The parts of a machine, such as a car engine, can also be described in different ways. One can just describe them in terms of configurations of parts and in terms of various relations between these parts. But one can also describe the elements of a machine in terms of what they can do or have a propensity to do. Is the latter some kind of 'mental' description of the machine?

This observation shows that the analysis of intentions in terms of propensities for action cannot be a complete analysis of their mental nature. (Observe, though, that some philosophers have believed that a dispositional analysis, or a neural state analysis coupled with a dispositional analysis, is all that is needed (Ryle 1949; Armstrong 1968).) My answer goes further. To have an intention is not just to have a disposition to act, it is also to have a disposition for some degree of awareness. If one intends one is disposed to believe that one intends, and also disposed to be aware of one's intention. Awareness itself cannot, I believe, be fully reduced to an action disposition. But on this point I will not try to pursue the analysis further.

Return now to actions and their analysis. The paradigm cases of action exist thus when persons who have formed an intention to do *F* – or decided to do *F*, which comes to the same thing – set themselves to do *F*. The intention underlying the action is often, but not always, conscious to the subjects. When I intend to travel to a place I am often aware of this. It is typical that I am highly aware of it at the moment of decision, i.e. the moment when I form my intention. But crucial exceptions occur. The existence of unconscious intentions was particularly forcefully stressed by Sigmund Freud (1915/1957) in his theory of psychoanalysis. It is also common knowledge that people who perform such actions, as have become automatized, are not always conscious of the intentions behind these actions. Consider, for instance, the complicated action-sequence involved in the driving of a car. Drivers are not always conscious of their intentions when they move the wheel. Nor are they continuously conscious of what direction they are going in. Nevertheless, the driving is almost always intentional.

Another case where the intention is not normally conscious is the case of an immediate reaction to an unexpected external event. A person who observes a car moving at high speed in his or her direction and immediately reacts by jumping aside does not consciously form an intention to jump. The action is more like a reflex movement. Nevertheless, it is obviously not a reflex proper. It is highly different from the patellar reflex, for instance. The patellar reflex, in order to release, does not depend on any cognition on the part of the subject. The subject does not have to observe anything. This is necessary, however, in the case of the person in traffic. The person notices the approaching car and intentionally jumps aside, although he or she is not aware, indeed has no time to be aware, of the working of the intentional mechanism.

I have equated a decision with the formation of an intention. When I decide to go to my job I form the intention to do this. I do not wish to presuppose, though, that a decision is the only way by which an intention can come about. For a further discussion about this, see Chapter 3 on mental abilities.

1.4 A modern theory of mind and matter

One can ask further questions about the mental propensity that constitutes an intention. What is the basis of it? Does a physical, say neurological, basis exist for every intention? On this issue there is a vast philosophical and scientific literature. Several treatments during the last 40 years have proposed a so-called materialistic theory of the mind (one of the earlier ones was Armstrong 1968). Such a theory involves the idea that an intention (as a mental state) is actually identical with a neurological (or in general physical) state. This proposal can be developed in two ways. The extreme interpretation is that there is a type-type relationship between the mental state and the neurological one. By this is meant that an intention of the type: A intends to go home, is identical with a type of neurological phenomenon situated in a particular part of the brain. Another, more plausible, interpretation proposes a token-token relationship. By this is meant that for every instance of the intention of type: A intends to go home, there is some neurological state with which the intention-instance is identical. One reason why this is a more plausible analysis of the relation between mind and matter is that it is common knowledge that the brain is plastic and that different parts of the brain can substitute for each other under special circumstances. A person who has lost a mental capacity in an accident, for instance the capacity to talk, can often regain this capacity although the damaged part of the brain is never reconstructed. Another part of the brain does the job of the old part. This observation opens the door to the possibility that a particular intention could be materially realized by slightly different neural events or states.

This plausible suggestion about some kind of identity between mental and neural states encounters, however, serious problems. One of the fundamental problems concerns a feature that is typical for mental states. A mental state, such as a perception, an intention or an emotion, is *directed towards something*, an object or a state of affairs, which is typically situated outside the person him- or herself. The person perceives *something*, intends to perform *an action*, or is happy or angry concerning *something*. In short, the states of the mind are *about something* and how could this feature be materialized in the brain. Our ordinary biological descriptions do not reflect this aboutness.

There is an enormous philosophical literature trying to solve the conundrums about the relation between body and mind. (For a distinguished overview, see Heil and Mele 1993.) This is not the place to review this discussion. For my own purposes I will ally myself with a recent very impressive attempt to analyse this relation, namely Bolton and Hill (2003). (For a brief introduction, see Bolton 2003.) This analysis also draws conclusions with regard to the explanation of mental illness. Presenting the plausible intuitions (1) that mental and neural events ought to stand in a close relation to each other and (2) that mental events must have a causal capacity and be able to influence events in the subject's body as well as in the external world, Bolton and Hill seek to reconcile them with the observation that our mental concepts have features that are so different from our biological concepts. Their solution relies on the idea that mental states are in fact 'encoded' in neural states. Neural states encode and process information. And, Bolton and Hill say, there is a biological language for describing information processing. This gives the identity theory a different and more sophisticated twist. Indeed, Bolton and Hill abstain from using the term 'identity theory'. The mental events are not, they say, identical with the neural events. They are 'realized' in neural events.

What does it mean to say that a mental event is encoded in the brain? Can we say this without just applying the mentalistic language to neural events? This can be seen more clearly if we replace the traditional biological language with another language, still within the framework of science, that emphasizes biological function rather than static properties.

According to Bolton and Hill, and with this I agree, what is typical for our mental states is that they are action-oriented. This is evidently so with wants and intentions, which are directly action-oriented. But it also holds for, for instance, cognitions and emotions. Cognitions and emotions are results of the person's confrontations with reality but the person does not just store these cognitions or emotions without any purpose. These states are parts of the continuous steering mechanisms in our lives. And our lives by and large consist of actions, actions for survival and actions for self-realization.

The 'encoding' of mental states could thus be described in the following way. When a man has the intention to walk home from his work, he has in his brain an encoded structure. This structure contains a causal mechanism to the effect that certain muscles, mainly in his legs, are triggered so that they finally issue in walking behaviour. This causal mechanism can in principle be formulated in purely biological terms. But since these terms are functional and causal, pointing to external effects, they can fulfil the crucial requirement of 'about-ness' that our mental concepts presuppose. The intentional description is forward-looking and action- oriented. In this case the biological description is also forward-looking and behaviour-oriented.

Given this functional twist in the biological description, it is natural to endorse a token-token variant of identity theory. John's intention to go home need not be realized in a very particular region of the brain. As long as the neural causal struc-ture is devised as it should, we do not require that particular nerve cells should be involved in the structure. I quote from Bolton and Hill (2003, p. 61):

> The question under consideration is whether from the external point of view, in the context of explaining behaviour in terms of mental states, these states can be identi-fied with material states of the brain. The answer is that it is possible, provided that the latter are described in terms of informational content and processing. If, on the

other hand, neural states and processes are described in a lower-level, non-intentional language, without reference to information, then it is a mistake to make the identification, for an essential feature of mental states is not captured in these lower-level descriptions.

And they go on to say on p. 62:

According to this argument, the valid sense of 'identity' here would have to be that in which functional states are 'realized by', 'served by', or 'implemented by' material processes.

It is evident that Bolton and Hill's solution squares very well with the general dispositional analysis of intentions that I have already indicated and will explore further in this book. I can now paraphrase this analysis in the following way: When a person has an intention he or she is in a neural state that is such that the person has a propensity for acting in a certain way. This is not indeed to say that the neural state is the 'same thing' as the mental state. Nor is it so say that a one-to-one correspondence exists between a type of neural state and a type of mental state. A crucial ingredient in an intention, as I have said, is its referential nature. An intention is an intention to act or to reach a goal. An identifying description of an intention requires a reference to an action or a further goal. In order to identify an intention with a particular structure in a brain, we must be able to identify this structure as a causal mechanism directed towards a certain kind of behaviour.

1.5 Actions and descriptions: the relation between intentions and actions

What is the relation between an intention and the action issuing from it? Is there a one-to-one relationship in the sense that the action F must issue from the intention to do F and no other intention? This is a highly complex issue and has to do with the ways by which we identify both intentions and actions. I will return to this in Sections 1.6, 1.7, and 1.11. Here, I will only note that accepted ways exist for identifying an intentional action F that need not relate to the intention to F. What is normally needed, however, is that some intention exists which is related to the action performed. A young boy may intend to score a goal when he is playing football. Unfortunately, however, the ball smashes a window of a nearby house. The action that he has performed would be recognized as his smashing the window. The boy would normally be held accountable for the action of smashing the window although it was never his intention to act in this way. His smashing of the window is still considered to be an action, since there was *some* intention behind his doing, namely the intention to kick the ball towards the goal.

The choice of intention as the distinguishing criterion of action is a natural and common one, but it is not the only possible choice. The law must for some purposes use a slightly wider notion of action than we normally recognize. The concept of *responsibility* is the crucial concept in the legal context. Everything for which an agent could be held responsible is an action performed by the agent. This may include certain cases of negligence and of omission. Although most instances of negligence and omission can be identified under some other intentional action description, as in the smashing-the-window case, this is not always so. Thus, the criterion of responsibility used in the legal context covers almost but not completely the same area as the criterion of intention. I will in the following stick to the criterion of intention.

Let me return to the question about the relation between actions and intentions. So far I have said that an intention to perform F (or some other intention) issues in an action. There is an intention (conscious or unconscious) existing for some time before the occurrence of a piece of behaviour and standing in a certain relation to the behaviour. What kind of relation is this? Is it causal in the way that an intention is an entity independent of the subsequent action and which causes this action? Or is the intention rather an integral part of the action? These questions have given rise to a great controversy in modern theory of action. The answers to them are of great importance for one's view of human beings and thereby for the theory of the disciplines studying human beings, namely the humanities. Are human beings essentially like machines and can they be understood as such? Or are they peculiar creatures that require special methods to be understood?

In a later section I will attempt to show that an intention is neither a cause of an action nor an integral part of an action. However, I would say that an intention *enters into* a causal explanation of action. It plays much the same part in such a causal explanation as a disposition plays. For most purposes the intention must be understood as something independent of the action. It is possible to hold this thesis and at the same time hold that the concept of action requires the concept of intention. To illustrate this possibility consider the following. Many species of diseases are defined in terms of their causes. The disease of tuberculosis, for instance, is defined as a kind of infection that is caused by *Mycobacterium tuberculosum*. The infection is clearly a process distinct from the occurrence of the mycobacterium. However, a particular infection would not be identified as an instance of tuberculosis unless it were caused by the right bacillus. Similarly, a bodily movement is not an action unless a causal explanation of the bodily movement exists, where an intention plays a certain role.

1.6 **Action-types and action-instances**

Cooking one's meal and running a marathon are two examples of action-types. John's cooking his evening meal at 6 o'clock on 7 July 1997, is an action-instance.

The same distinction can be made in the world of objects. A book is an object-type; the book that lies on my table now is an instance of this type of object. The things, as well as the events and actions, that we observe in the world are all instances. Types are abstractions that we need in order to understand and organize the elements of the world.

Types can vary from being extremely general to being extremely specific. If we wished we could organize the whole universe of actions in trees of orders, classes, families, genera, and species in the way Linnaeus and others have organized the biological world. 'Acting' would then itself be the most general of all action-types. 'Cooking' is a type on the medium level; 'cooking dinner' is a more specific version; 'cooking dinner in a French style with red wine' is quite a specific type, but it can be made much more specific. If we try very hard we can create an action-type so specific that it can in practice have only one instance. But we must remember, a description becomes a description of an action-instance and not of a type as soon as we add exact time and space parameters: 'John's cooking dinner in his own kitchen at 6 o'clock on 7 July 1997' is a description of an action-instance and not of a specific action-type. Observe also that the description of an action-instance need not be very specific. 'There is now some cooking being performed in this kitchen' is a description of an action-instance.

It is important to keep in mind the difference between general and specific action-types, as well as the distinction between types and instances. In having the former distinction in mind one avoids, for instance, the confusion of regarding cooking as an action that is different from cooking a meal. This is a confusion that is similar to regarding a seabird as something different from a gull. Cooking a meal is a species of cooking in the same way as a gull is a species of seabird.

1.7 Actions under different descriptions

Given the observations above, it is evident that one and the same action-instance can be described in many ways. It can be described very generally and very specifically. No limits exist for describing it. This can seem disturbing. Can one not find a privileged way of describing an action-instance, a way that is better than other possible ways of identifying this particular action-instance? Is 'some cooking now being performed in the kitchen' a description that is as adequate as 'John is now cooking veal together with peas, carrots, and potatoes in the kitchen?' All our intuitions tell us that the latter description is superior. One reason for this is that it is the more informative description. But is the most informative (true) description necessarily the most adequate one? Is that description of John's action best which tells us all possible details about his cooking: for instance, how much water he has in his saucepan, how many ounces of spices he has, how long it takes for the water to boil, etc.? We realize that this cannot in general be the case.

My suggestion is that one description of an action-instance exists which – in most cases – has a privileged status. This is the description which best matches John's intention in his acting. If John intended to cook his veal with carrots, peas, and potatoes and nothing more specific, then this description is – for most purposes – the most adequate description of his subsequent action. And if we ask what type of action John has performed an instance of, then the type should ultimately be identified with the help of the description which best matches his intention. (I shall develop this point further in a later section.) An important presupposition here, however, is that John is not prevented from performing the action in the way he intended. One can imagine the case where John intends to travel to Mumbai by air, but as there is a hurricane preventing the plane from landing in Mumbai, John ends up in Delhi. His action can then hardly be identified as 'travelling to Mumbai', at most it can be described as 'attempting to travel to Mumbai'. One can say that there is a complete match between intentions and subsequent attempts to act in a certain way.

Again in some legal cases, action descriptions exist which are considered adequate for the legal purpose but which are not identical with the action description that would best fit the agent's own intentions. A burglar who is entering a house to grab some jewellery would hardly him- or herself classify the action as an instance of burglary but simply as the action of getting hold of the valuable stuff in the house that he or she has entered.

Before proceeding, I will add a note on terminology. Although I have emphasized the importance of the distinction between action-types and action-instances, I will in the following not always mark that distinction in the text. To avoid awkwardness in style I will, for instance, use the ordinary phrase 'to perform an action' instead of the clumsy but correct 'to perform an instance of an action-type'.

1.8 **From simple actions to complex actions**

We can find an enormous variety of actions, from the simplest to the most complicated ones. Some actions involve only the intentional movement of a part of the body, for instance the movement of a finger. Other actions entail that the agent creates something or performs some reorganization in the external world, for instance in building a house. Yet other actions presuppose the existence of a society with its bureaucratic and legal structure; this is, for example, true of the action of sentencing a criminal to imprisonment.

We can look at these matters more systematically. What further things than a bodily movement can be involved in an action? Let me here mention some salient factors and give examples. I will then divide the universe of actions into *natural actions* and *conventional actions*, two concepts that will be further considered below.

Factors which could be involved in natural actions apart from a series of bodily movements are the following:

- a physical object: knock on a door
- a tool plus a physical object: sweep a floor
- an object plus a tool plus a change in the object: paint a wall
- an object plus a change in the object's relations to other objects: open a door
- objects and tools plus the creation of a new object: build a house
- an object plus the destruction of the object: pull down a house, eat food
- an object plus the prevention of a result: keep the enemy at bay

The four latter kinds of actions have in common that they entail a particular *result or its prevention* in the external world. This is a feature that is typical for most action-types.

A conventional action is an action that presupposes the existence of a rule laid down by society or some part of society, in the limiting case by the agent him- or herself. Such a rule is of the following kind: an intentional physical movement of type M should in circumstances C be counted as an action of type T. Two examples are these: lifting one's hat when meeting a person counts as greeting this person; making certain laryngeal noises modified by certain lip-movements in a certain sequence counts as speaking a language. The rule used here is of the *constitutive* kind. (See Searle 1969, for this term.) Constitutive rules must be distinguished from *regulative* rules to be introduced below.

It is salient that the use of language plays an enormous role in the 'creation' of conventional actions. Consider the following central variants of actions and activities that presuppose the existence of language:

- the existence of language: give information
- the existence of language and the existence of a rule-governed activity, for instance a game: play cards
- the existence of language and the existence of institutions: open a bank account
- the previous conditions plus the presence of other persons: sentence a criminal to imprisonment.

The conventional action of marrying another person is a classical example of a conventional action with many presuppositions. Marrying presupposes: the existence of the institution of matrimony, the fact that the event has been previously announced, the presence of a partner, the presence of a priest (or equivalent person), the presence of witnesses, some actions performed by the priest according to a ritual, and the subsequent language acts performed by the two partners according to the ritual. See Austin (1975) for the classical presentation of this example.

Most conventional actions also entail results. These results, however, are all results in the conventional world. The following are two examples. The existence of a bank account is the conventional result of opening a bank account. The existence of a marriage between a man and a woman is a result of the action of marrying.

1.9 **Actions: their results and consequences**

I noted above that many actions entail results. An action-concept typically indicates the result of the action instead of the process that leads up to the result. Consider all the following examples of actions: close a door, create an object, destroy an object, kill a person, complete a project, take an exam, appoint a president. In all these cases the action-concept points at the final result rather than the activity that has to be performed to reach the result. In some action-theoretic analyses such concepts have been called *act-concepts* and the actions signified have been called *acts*.

Georg Henrik von Wright has created a logical theory of acts. He analyses an act as a change in the world that has been brought about by an agent. The agent *A* has performed an act when he or she has changed the world from an initial state *non-p* to a final state *p*. von Wright (1963) proposes the following formalism for this statement: *Do (non-p T p)*. The whole focus in von Wright's formalization of acts, then, is on the change in the world. There is no place for the bodily movements of the agent in this picture. von Wright's idea seems plausible, however, if the purpose is to analyse the ordinary *act-concepts*. The ordinary concept of closing a door, for instance, does not refer to anything but the change in the world. It does not say whether the agent brought about this change by means of his or her hands, legs, or the whole body, or for that matter, by means of blowing at the door.

But not all actions are of the act kind. Some actions are *activities*. Walking is an activity and playing with a ball is an activity. The concept of walking points at what is going on, viz. that the agent moves his or her feet on the ground in moving forwards. Playing with a ball is a bit more abstract, but it likewise indicates that the agent is in the process of touching a ball with his or her hands, legs, or some other part of the body. The concept does not, however, point to any end. There is nothing in the concept of walking which says when the action will be terminated, nor is there anything in the concept of playing that indicates what constitutes the termination of playing.

Aristotle was quite aware of these different kinds of doing. He called the activities *energeiai* ('actualities' as the term is normally translated) and the acts *kineseis* ('movements' and 'doings' are typical translations). These terms also covered non-intentional doings. This is easily seen when we consider some of the verb-types that signify non-intentional doings or happenings in the world. 'Sleeping' is an *energeia*. It is a state that does not point to an end. Sleeping can, as far as the concept is concerned, go on indefinitely. 'Splitting' is a *kinesis*. Splitting can indeed be an intentional action but also a natural happening as in 'the lightning split the tree'.

Aristotle made the interesting observation that different logical relations exist between the tenses of the verbs denoting activities and acts. 'At the same time we are thinking and have thought, while it is not true that at the same time we are learning and have learnt, or are being cured and have been cured' (*Metaphysics* 1048 b.) Or, to illustrate the same idea with other examples: when we say that John is playing it must also hold true that John has already played (for some period of time), but when we say that John is closing the door it is untrue to say that he has closed the door. This is of course due to the fact that an activity is an action that *lasts for* some time. An act does not last for some time. An act may *take* some time to complete, but it can also be instantaneous. (The latter, instantaneous kinds of acts, were labelled by Gilbert Ryle 1949 as 'achievements'.)

Also modern linguistic philosophers and grammarians have noted similar differences between activity-verbs and act-verbs. They have formalized grammatical tests by which one can distinguish between the two kinds. For act-verbs the following is assumed to hold: *A* is *F-ing* only if *A* has not *F-ed*. For activity-verbs the implication is instead: *A* is *F-ing* only if *A* has *F-ed*. Examples: *A* is killing Mr Smith, implies that *A* has not yet killed Mr Smith. But: *A* is now playing with the ball, implies: *A* has played with the ball for some time. (For further details and complications in these relations, see Kenny 1963, Vendler 1967, and Nordenfelt 2000.)

I have said that acts are identified by their *results*, which terminate the action. The result is in a way included in the act. When the result has been achieved the act can no longer go on. Results as included in their actions should, however, be distinguished from the *consequences* of actions. All actions, including activities, have consequences that are for the most part unintended by the agent. A consequence of one's walking may be that one gets tired, a consequence of one's playing with a ball may be that one finds a new friend. And a consequence of closing the door may be that one makes a terrible noise.

The results of acts, as I have said, define when the acts have come to an end. To complicate the story we can see that also some activities have results (if we press the point perhaps *all* activities), in the sense that a change in the world can be entailed by the activity-concept itself. Torturing is an example. When an agent is torturing another person then it is entailed that the latter is in pain. If the activity performed does not have pain as a result then it cannot be an act of torturing. However, torturing is still an activity. The resulting pain does not terminate the action in question. The action of torturing can go on indefinitely.

In the case where the consequences of one action are intended, these consequences are normally the intended results of a further action planned by the agent. This observation brings us to the topic of hierarchies of actions and the phenomenon of action-generation.

1.10 **On complexes of actions**

Human beings are sometimes rational agents who plan their lives. They may even make fairly long-term plans entailing sequences of actions in order to reach a goal. Suppose that we have a person who wishes to take a university degree. In order to reach this goal the agent has to take examinations in a number of subjects, say politics, economics, and philosophy. Thus the person must first read politics, then economics and then philosophy. This preliminary division can be made even more fine-grained. Studying politics may entail reading a certain number of books and writing a certain number of papers. This in its turn can be further divided into simpler actions and action-sequences.

In a way we can then say that we have a hierarchy of actions. On the top of the hierarchy we have the grand action of taking a university degree. Below that we have the actions of studying politics, economics, and philosophy. Below these in their turn we have a further set of actions. This hierarchical relation is in ordinary language often indicated by two kinds of locution. The choice of one or the other depends on the perspective from which one looks upon the relation. If we look upon it from the perspective of the agents when they initiate the action-sequence we use the locution 'in order to'. The agents read books in economics in order to take an examination in economics. They take this examination in order to complete their degree. The locution 'in order to' indicates that the agent has more than one intention in performing his or her action. I will study this more closely in the section about intention transmission.

But if we look upon the hierarchy from the perspective of the completed action we can use the locution 'by doing'. The agents complete their degree *by* taking an examination in economics. They pass their examination in economics by studying hard, etc. (Observe that the by-locution does not in itself indicate agency; see Bennett 1988.)

Two fundamental mechanisms exist by means of which we can construct hierarchies of actions. One mechanism entails making *sequences of actions,* i.e. performing one action after another. The other mechanism entails the use of the external world and its causal and conventional machinery. In the latter construction of a hierarchy of actions there is in fact only one so-called *basic action* needed, namely one intentional bodily movement. The rest is produced by the environment. I will explain this phenomenon.

Consider the following example. John starts the car by twisting a key in the ignition. John twists the key in its turn by turning his hand rightwards. In this case we have only one basic action, viz. one intentional bodily movement. But at the same time at least two other actions are performed, the twisting of the key and the starting of the car. Through the bodily movement a part of the external world is changed and a causal chain has been initiated. When the key is moved in the ignition there is an electrical circuit closed, which has as its effect that the engine of the car starts. The basic action in question has *generated* two other actions. (For a detailed account of the notion of action generation, see Goldman 1970.)

The mechanism behind the generation in my example was causal. The hand movement caused a number of subsequent states of affairs. This kind of generation is typical. This is what is involved in all actions that entail the creation of a new state of affairs in the physical world, i.e. in most of the act-types as analysed by von Wright. However, causation – at least as understood physically – is not the only mechanism of generation available. We can also conceive of *conventional* generation. By this we mean the case when a person, for instance, by writing his or her name according to conventional rules can create a great number of different other actions, such as establishing a contract, opening a bank account or buying a house. (See the account of the concept of conventional action above.) In such a case there is also just one basic action involved, the movement of one's hand in writing. The rest is effected through the external 'conventional' world.

The series of actions that come into being through action-generation will in the following be called *action-chains*, as distinguished from *action-sequences*. A good example of an action-sequence can be taken from our study-example. In reading one book after another in economics, the person performs a multitude of basic actions: picking up the first book, sitting down, reading page one, turning to page two, reading page two, etc. It is typical that action-sequences take a long time to reach the final goal, in this case the degree.

Most action-sequences also involve action-chains. Many of the elements in an action-sequence involve the manipulation of the external world in one way or the other. Picking up a book, for instance, is not, strictly speaking, a basic action. The basic action involved is lifting one's hand. This means that most action-sequences are complex in two ways.

I introduced this section by saying that people are at least occasionally rational and plan their lives. This entails that they set up goals for their actions. In many cases the goals are quite precise end-states. Such end-states are marked by act-verbs such as 'closing a door', 'killing a person', and 'taking an exam'. In many cases the goal can be reached through one basic action, for instance a quick movement of one's hand. In other cases, reaching the goal requires a compli-cated action-sequence, as in taking an exam. The action-chain that leads up to the end-state I shall call an *accomplishment*. The action-sequence that leads up to a final goal I shall call a *project*. (For a similar theory, refer to the work by the Russian psychologist Aleksei Leontiev 1981.)

Not all action-chains and action-sequences terminate in a definite end-state. In some cases the ultimately generated action is an activity. From this does not follow, however, that it is purposeless. Some activities are of a maintenance character. The purpose of the activity could be to keep something going, perhaps indefinitely. A worker in an industry may have as his duty to see to it that certain engines keep going, that they never stop. This activity of monitor-ing the engines may entail both action-chains and action-sequences which in themselves may or may not have definite terminating end-states, but the monitoring itself – which is definitely an action-sequence – has no terminat-ing end-state. Thus, the activity of monitoring is not a project in my sense.

1.11 On the individuation of action-instances and of action-types

Here, I have considered a great multiplicity of actions. Basic actions can gener-ate higher-order actions and form accomplishments. Accomplishments can in their turn form sequences of actions and end up in projects. I have also, following another ground for division, distinguished between activities and acts. I have furthermore noted how actions can be described in different ways. One can then wonder how actions can be individuated. When can we claim that two actions are identical with another? When do people perform the same actions?

The question about individuation of actions can be asked on two levels, the level of action-instances and the level of action-types. Let me start on the level of types. I shall concentrate on the case where two action-instances can be said to belong to *the same type of action*. The number of action-types is very great and open-ended. We create new action-types all the time, for instance by installing new institutions and creating new technologies. Think of all the new actions that have been introduced through the IT revolution. The action language is continuously growing.

The number of action-types is very great also because of all of their possible combinations that I have just indicated. One can perform F by performing $F1$ and $F2$. But one can also perform F by performing $F3$ and $F4$. Moreover, both $F2$ and $F4$ may be performed in different ways, etc. The complex F $(By\ F1,\ F2)$ is an action-type that is different from the complex F $(By\ F3,\ F4)$. Thus, a person who is performing the first complex and another person who is performing the latter complex are performing two different types of action.

I will illustrate this case. Both John and Peter are stealing a car. John, however, is stealing his car by manipulating documents concerning the ownership of the car. Peter, on the other hand, is stealing his car by physically breaking into the car. According to this reasoning, then, they are performing actions of different types.

But is it possible, then, for two people to perform an action of the same type? Can we not always find minute differences between two actions such that the actions could be counted as instances of two distinct types? My answer is that, although ultimately most action-instances are of different types, it is possible for two people to perform an action of the same type. One must not confuse the open-endedness of all possible true descriptions of actions with the open-endedness of all true action-identifying descriptions. One can always find some difference between the action that John is doing and the action that Peter is doing. John may be acting more quickly than Peter, or John may be acting more elegantly than Peter. However, these are not action-identifying differences *unless John*, in contradistinction to Peter, *has intended to act quickly or elegantly*. So if John has decided to steal a Volvo by breaking into it and has decided to break into it with the help of a jemmy, and subsequently sets about doing so, and Peter has decided to steal a Volvo by breaking into it and has decided to break into it with the help of a jemmy, and then sets about doing so, then John and Peter have performed an action of ultimately the same type. This is so even if John steals his Volvo in Coventry, does so in a clumsy way and uses a jemmy that is white, and Peter steals his Volvo in Birmingham, does so in an elegant way and uses a jemmy that is yellow. The latter properties of the action-instances in question were never intentional elements of the actions.

Now, we rarely have need of the notion of 'ultimately the same action-type'. We often need to be able to talk about the same action-type in a more preliminary way, a way that is sufficient for a certain purpose. In particular, there is a need in moral and legal theory to identify action-types on a level that is morally and legally relevant. This level is often of a high degree of generality. 'Stealing' is a level that is morally and legally relevant. But also the level of breaking into someone's property is morally and legally relevant. However, not all levels of intentionality are morally and legally relevant. If John and Peter both decide to use a jemmy of a certain brand, then these decisions are morally and legally irrelevant.

Now, is it disturbing that an action-instance can be said to belong to a great number of types? And is this something peculiar to the ontology of actions? I will consider the latter question first. The ontology of actions is not special in this respect. The traditional biological hierarchies are at least partly similar. The animal that I have in my garden is a bird, but it is also a duck as well as a duck of a particular type. It is true to say for some purposes that I and my neighbour have the same kind of animal when we say that we have a bird. But for another purpose we need to specify, and thereby find that we have different kinds of birds.

One can still say that actions are peculiar in the way that one action can be *embedded* in another kind of action, and that both can be subsumed under a third kind of action (in the way I have explained above). We say that John by crooking his finger fires his gun and by doing so wounds another person. One can maintain that this series is different from the biological hierarchy of animals or plants, in that the members of the action-chain incorporate lesser and greater chunks of reality. The crooking incorporates only the intentional bodily movement, the firing furthermore incorporates an event within the mechanism of the gun, and the wounding incorporates a change in another person's body.

Although the phenomenon of embedded actions in chains and sequences is typical for actions – which is the reason why I have dwelt upon it here – embeddedness of phenomena of the same ontological types as such is not peculiar to actions. It holds for the whole universe of events. A meteorite may kill a man by falling on him. The falling of the stone is embedded in the more inclusive event of killing the man. Consider also for the case of physical objects the example of Chinese boxes. Assume that there is a little ball in one of the smallest boxes. And assume that one asks in what box it is. There can be as many true answers as there are levels of boxes. All answers are true but not all of them are relevant for all purposes. It is also true here – as in the case of action-chains and action-sequences – that the biggest box incorporates a bigger part of reality than any of the lower-level boxes.

This reasoning concludes my answer to the question whether the indeterminateness of what action-type a particular action instance belongs to is a problem. This indeterminateness is no more disturbing than that which we find in other areas of reality. And this is not disturbing at all. It only provides us with a richness of means for identifying and talking about phenomena. Moreover, one can also say that the field of actions is less indeterminate than other fields. As I have indicated, a sense exists in which one can talk about the ultimately true action-type. This is the type indicated by the agent's own intentionality. If John intends to open the bathroom door (and nothing more), and then sets about doing so, then he has performed the action of opening the bathroom door.

So much for individuation of action-types and the criteria of sameness of action-types. Consider now individuation of action-instances. I have already mentioned instances, and part of the work of identifying types is also a matter of identifying instances. But I have not fully answered the question regarding individuating instances. When we say that John and Peter perform the same action then it is clear that we are talking about sameness of types. An action-instance can only have one agent. The agent, though, need not be an individual human being; it could be an institution or a collection of human beings.

The distinguishing feature of an instance is that it is an occurrence at a definite time and place. An instance of a physical object occupies a certain time and place. An event occurs at a definite time and place or within a definite period and within a definite region. The latter holds good also for actions. Moreover, in the case of actions there is one identified agent. It is therefore impossible to say that agent A is performing the same action-instance as agent B, unless A and B are identical or belong to the same collective, where, strictly speaking, the collective is the agent.

A few things have to be disentangled here. First, action-types *may* involve both times and places. They may also involve roughly the same times and places. John may intend to participate in the rowing race on the River Thames on 2 July 1999 at 14.00. Peter may intend to do the same thing; in fact they intend to compete in the same race. Assume that they actually do participate. Although the descriptions of what they are doing may be identical also in terms of time- and space-references, they clearly do not perform the same action-instances. John and Peter are different agents and a very specific description of the time and, in particular, the space that their actions occupy would show this clearly.

Second, we must return to the phenomenon of embeddedness and its relevance for the identification of action-instances. The crucial question is: Should we say that A's crooking his finger at time t and place p is the same action-instance as his shooting Smith at time t and place p? Or, are they different instances? One can say that there is one crucial reason for distinguishing between the two. A's shooting Smith incorporates, strictly speaking, a bigger chunk of reality than A's crooking his finger. Nature has to operate for a few seconds after the crooking of the finger until Smith is wounded and the action of shooting Smith has been completed. This reasoning indicates that the action-instance of A's wounding Smith at t–$t1$ and p–$p1$ includes the action-instance of A's crooking his finger at t and p. This is completely analogous to how a big box includes a small box.

Does a reason exist to the contrary, i.e. that the crooking and the wounding are one and the same instance? I think this is so and I will argue for that mode of speech. Unless we say that John's crooking his finger at t is the same instance as his wounding Smith at t–$t1$, we cannot easily express the fundamental difference between this case and the one when John crooks his finger and shoots at something, while at the same time in using his other hand he wounds Smith with a knife. In the latter case, John does two different things, he performs two different action-instances at the same time. In the other case John acts once, performs one basic action, which results in the wounding of Smith. And even if we were to describe the relation between a basic action and its generated actions as a part-whole relation, we have anyway thereby admitted that there is some numerical identity. A part is identical with the phenomenon of which it is a part. (See Goldman 1970, and Davidson 1981, for reasonings in the same direction.)

Summary concerning the locution 'the same action'. I have identified two major cases where it is reasonable to talk about sameness of actions. One case concerns sameness of types. John and Peter perform the same type of action if they successfully perform an action under the same intentional description. If John intends to steal a car, and does it, and Peter intends to steal a car, and does it, then they have performed the same type of action. The other case concerns sameness of instances. This can only hold for one and the same agent. John and Peter cannot perform the same action-instance. However, when John performs a generated action *F1* he must at the same time perform a basic action *F*. I have argued that *F* is a part of *F1* and thereby identical with *F1* in the part-whole sense.

1.12 **Actions that do not involve bodily movements**

I will add two more abstract classifications of some importance. Hitherto I have presupposed that all actions involve bodily movements of some kind. This is the standard case. We can, however, find two classes of actions for which this presupposition does not hold. These are *mental actions* and *omissions*.

To think, is at least often to perform an action. I can decide to think about my future or about action theory and then proceed to do so. These kinds of thinking thus fulfil the requirements of being actions. Although many people cannot think without using a pen or without talking to themselves, thinking need not, of course, involve a bodily movement. Therefore, there are action-types that do not presuppose any bodily movements. Thinking is a paradigm example of mental action having many subspecies such as fantasizing, day-dreaming, calculating, and analysing. There are, however, several other examples of mental actions, for instance looking and listening. I shall return to a more detailed discussion of mental actions and abilities below. (For a deeper analysis of mental actions, see Chapter 3, Section 3.2.)

A different but important class of actions that do not presuppose bodily movements is constituted by omissions. These are a kind of negative actions that are derivative of their positive counterparts. When one omits, one always omits to perform some specific positive act. For instance, a housekeeper omits to go to the shop or the doctor omits to introduce life-saving measures in a case where a patient is dying.

One can wonder how the absence of action can count as an action. The fundamental answer in this case, as with actions in general, is that omissions are actions when they are intentional. The housekeeper who decides to abstain from going to the shop and the doctor who likewise decides not to introduce any life-saving measures, are both abstaining intentionally from doing something. Hence, they are performing actions.

But not all not-doing counts as action. The person who does not intend to drive a car and therefore is not driving is not performing any action in relation to driving. Similarly, the person who does not do any work and has not considered doing any, is not abstaining from working, i.e. is not performing the action of omitting to work. From the point of view of the law, there is an exception to the latter case. If an employer legitimately requires some work to be performed by a man, who still does not perform this work, then from a legal point of view the man is omitting to work and can be punished for that. This may hold even if the agent does not intend to omit to do his work.

Both mental actions and omissions can function as basic actions in the formation of action-chains. One can solve a problem by thinking about it. And one can assist a woman by omitting to put obstacles in her way.

1.13 **Rational actions and norms of actions**

In introducing the notion of intention I took my starting point in the fact that humans are rational agents who plan their activities and form intentions in accordance with their plans. I shall now develop this platform a bit further and I can use some of the notions already introduced.

A typical situation involving planning is the following. A man wants to travel a long way, say from Stockholm to Tokyo. He finds it realistic to make a plan for such a journey. He has sufficient money and he has the time and opportunity for this journey. Thus, because he decides to go to Tokyo, he forms this intention. But the planning has hereby just started. The man must find out how to go there. Does more than one route exist? Can more than one airline take him to the destination? What are the preferable options? As a result of this whole consideration the man comes up with a plan for his flight. He has decided to take a plane from Stockholm to Frankfurt, another plane from Frankfurt to Hong Kong and, finally, one the last bit to Tokyo.

This means that the man's journey can be divided into parts and it also means that he forms more than one intention. First exists the original intention to travel to Tokyo; but as a result of the planning the man also acquires the intentions to go to Frankfurt and Hong Kong. As a result of his intention to go to Tokyo and his acquired belief that going via Frankfurt and Hong Kong is necessary in order to travel to Tokyo in the most expedient way, he acquires the derived intentions to go to Frankfurt and Hong Kong. This is the phenomenon of *intention transmission.*

Intention transmission does not stop at this stage. The man must take several measures in order to get to Frankfurt. He must get up in time in the morning, he must dress and have breakfast, and he must take the car to Stockholm's Arlanda Airport. In all of these cases intentions have to be formed and they are formed as a result of his higher-order intention to go to Frankfurt together with his considerations concerning necessary means to the end. We can see how this analysis can be pursued in much greater detail until we end up with the basic actions and the man's intentions to perform the basic actions. A gigantic intentional tree can be drawn, where the man's intention to go to Tokyo is on the top and his intention to raise his body (the first morning when he starts his journey) is on the bottom.

This tree represents a rational order in one sense of this word: let us call it the sense of *logical intention transmission.* I will in a later chapter analyse this rational order in much more detail. It is crucial to observe that one and the same basic action can issue from different intentional trees. The man's intention to travel to Tokyo can exist parallel to his intention to see to his family's meal. For both purposes he must raise his body in order to deal with further matters. Thus, we here have a sense where a basic action can be intentionally over-determined.

Another sense of rationality presupposes that *good reasons* exist for forming the intention on the top level of the hierarchy. So far we have only assumed that the man wanted to travel to Tokyo. A further question to ask is whether he had good reasons for having this want and therefore for pursuing the journey. Such good reasons can be of various kinds. One kind of good reason is to see whether a journey to Tokyo fits well into the agent's general life-plan, for instance is in accord with what he otherwise wants to achieve professionally and privately. The journey is rational, i.e. the intention to travel to Tokyo is rational, if it supports or at least does not interfere with the other top-level wants that the man has. I will call this variety of good reasons the *coherence* sense.

A crucial variant of rationality relates the agent's intention to society. This is the rationality that means that a planned action is in accord with a societal *norm.* A norm states that a certain action is prescribed. It may say: In situation C the action to be performed is F. In this case the norm has the form of an obligation. The other main variants of norms are permissions: In situation C it is permitted to do F, and prohibitions: In situation C it is forbidden to do F.

From a material point of view, norms can be of various kinds and of various levels of significance. The most binding norms are the laws of a society; on a lower level we have rules issued by authorities positioned along a hierarchy of superiority. Among these rules we find traffic rules and rules of conduct in schools and other institutions. Such rules are proper rules in the sense that they are unconditional with regard to the agent's wants.

Outside the proper rules, one can find recommendations of a technical kind that are sometimes called rules. A recipe in a cook book contains such technical rules. It may say: when you bake a strawberry cake for four persons, you should have two eggs in the dough. This is a quasi-rule since it presupposes that the agent wants to bake a strawberry cake; moreover there is no real obligation to follow the rule. The author of the recipe only conveys a piece of information that may play a role in the intention transmission of the reader: If you follow my recommendation you will get a cake that is nice and tasty.

In what sense do norms have anything to do with rationality? This question has a number of answers. First, society itself in terms of its legislating institutions normally considers the norm itself to be rational. In the best of worlds, society has good reasons for instituting its norms. Here, society can be considered to be a collective agent that should give good reasons for its norms. These good reasons should ultimately be given in coherence terms. A norm must be part of a plan that should not interfere with any other important plan that the society has. If the norm is rational in this way (from a societal point of view), one may say that a citizen who infringes it is irrational irrespective of the citizen's own wants and judgments.

A particular agent can have good reasons for following a norm that are more individual. These reasons are typically connected with some high-order wants of the agent. Two salient reasons of this type are the following. The agent wants to be a member of the society in question. He or she finds that it is not possible in the long run to remain a member of the society unless one follows (most of) the rules laid down by its legislating bodies. The rationality then exists in terms of coherence between the agent's want to follow some norms and his or her want to remain a member of the society. A second highly concrete reason can be the agent's want to avoid the sanctions that typically follow from the breaking of a rule. For instance, in order to avoid a severe traffic penalty, a driver must not exceed 60 miles an hour on the highway.

For a more comprehensive analysis of the notion of rational action, see Chapter 5.

1.14 **To perform an action and to perform an action well**

In many cases, not least in the context of health care, there is a need for distinguishing between performing an action and performing an action well.

Situations exist when it is important to perform an action well. A father tells his son to wash himself properly. Or a teacher tells a student to perform well during a course so that she will get her degree. But what do 'goodness' and similar terms refer to here? There is a battery of distinctions to be made.

1.14.1 Doing F and not-doing F

We must first become clear about the distinction between when the agent really has performed F and when he or she has not performed F at all. This distinction is fairly clear when we deal with acts. Acts, as I said, have results. An act is not completed unless the result has become the case. One has not closed the door unless there is a door that is closed. One has not passed an exam unless there is a final document proving it. So the result's being there and the agent's being, through an intentional doing of his or hers, causally responsible for the result, is a sufficient criterion of the act's having been performed.

But what about activities? Some activities have results, although, per definition, not terminating results. To be torturing a person is to be involved in an activity that conceptually entails that somebody else is in pain. If the result is not there or is not continuously there, the agent is no longer torturing. If one stretches the notion of result one can perhaps say that most activities entail some continuous result. (It is even possible to view the entailed bodily movements as a result of the activity.) The activity of reading entails a certain up-take on the part of the agent. If people do not absorb the text in question or do not understand what is read then they are not really reading. The activity of walking can perhaps be analysed in a similar way. If the movement of the person's legs does not result in the movement of the whole body, then there is no walking. The entailed result is not there.

But this conclusion is problematic. Results are not always clearly defined. Closing a door and passing an exam appear to be the best-defined examples. In the latter case this can be accomplished through conventional stipulation. But what about: arriving in a town, baking a cake, and, in particular, the activity cases: reading, walking, and such a complex activity as administering a county council?

A woman can be arriving in a city in the sense that she has passed its borders. But that may perhaps not entail what was expected in the context; she may have been expected to arrive at the city centre. A trainee baker may be trying to bake a cake and he or she may produce something that is edible. Doubts can arise, however, as to whether most people would call the result a cake. And how much of a proper result should we require from the activities of reading and walking? How much should a person understand in order to be accepted as reading? How much should a person be able to move his or her legs in order to be labelled as walking? Consider the activity of administering a county council. How many decisions should be made? How many meetings should be held? These are genuine indeterminacies and they can only be answered by the introduction of *standards for performing the actions in question.*

1.14.2 **Standards for doing F**

Different standards exist. I will first consider the basic idea of a standard by which one can say whether an action has been performed at all. As I noted in the case of passing an exam, a number of legally formalized conventional actions exist, where *the results as well as other required circumstances* are clearly stipulated in a formal definition of the action. The reasons for these stipulations are obvious. No doubt shall exist concerning when a couple is married, when a criminal has been sentenced, or when a will has become valid. Thus, such actions and their entailed results are defined as precisely as a human being can do. Moreover, when there is a lack of clarity this is normally straightened out by a court decision.

People may, however, perform other conventional actions where the result is unclear. When can I say that I have informed a person or warned a person? Do we require that this person has really heard and really understood my message? Or do we only require that I should have good reason to believe that the person has heard and understood? And, as we have seen with the above examples concerning different natural actions, no standard for judging when the required result has been achieved seems to exist.

The areas where standards have been well developed are law, administration, and medicine. Minimal requirements exist, for instance, for a county councillor. These are formulated in written instructions. If the instructions are not followed, the councillor is not really performing the job. To some extent health care institutions, in particular institutions of rehabilitation, have introduced standards for judging when a patient can be said to be doing such things as walking, talking, and reading. Such standards are necessary in order to define the rehabilitating tasks. It is necessary to ask such questions as: What is the goal of the rehabilitation of this man who cannot walk?

One efficient way of defining an action is to specify it as an act, i.e. specify a salient terminating result. In the case of the activity of walking this specification can be done by suggesting that the patients should be able to walk to the nearest shop, or that they should be able to walk up the stairs in their houses. Or, in the case of the activity of talking, the patients should be able to produce a short understandable message with their own voices. If such an end-result can be achieved then the agent can be said to have performed the action of talking.

This is not the only way of specifying an activity. One could, for instance, define walking in terms of how high one lifts one's legs or what distance forwards one is able to go with each step.

An interesting difference in character exists between the legal/administrative standard and the medical standard. In the former case no doubt can come up as to whether the agent is able to do what is required; the question is rather whether he or she is willing to do it. In the medical case the whole focus is on the agent's ability. The former standard is there to enforce action, and if it is not done, to hold a person legally responsible. The medical standard is there to help health care personnel in their efforts to rehabilitate patients.

1.14.3 Standards for action and standards for proper action

My focus has so far been completely on the basic criteria for the occurrence of an action of a certain type. Under what conditions has a person closed a door, baked a cake, passed an exam, walked, talked or administered a county council? I have said that the answer to this question frequently requires the introduction of a standard. This holds not only for the set of conventional actions (where this must be done almost per definition) but also for many natural actions, in particular natural activities. The notion of a standard, however, has a ring of *normativity* about it. Our initial task, however, was factual. We wanted to know about the existence conditions for actions. How should this be settled?

In one sense the normativity about standards is no problem or at least no exception in relation to, for instance, what is the case in science. We certainly talk about standards in many scientific contexts. For the purpose of exact measurement, for instance, one has to introduce standards to be followed all over the world. There is, for instance, a standard metre, situated in Paris, which stipulates the notion of a metre. There are thousands of other stipulated definitions in science. One has to follow these stipulations in order to be talking the scientific language correctly. Thus, on this level there is nothing particularly problematic about the action language.

But this is not the only normativity that is at stake in the case of action. The standard suggested for the county council administrators does not just tell us what are to be counted as actions or performance in their job. It also tells us what they are supposed to do as administrators. The instructions do not just contain constitutive rules for actions but also regulative rules, to speak as John Searle (1969) does. Or, the rules are at the same time constitutive and regulative. Not all of them need have this double function, of course. There may, for instance, be a lot of actions that are optional for the administrator. This double function of rules is common in the case of conventional actions. It is easy to illustrate this ambivalence from the field of games. The game of chess contains a number of constitutive rules, rules that define the different moves, and also what moves can be made in what order. If a player does something that is not defined, this move is no move at all, no action at all within the game. But apart from being no move this non-action, which is still an action in the ordinary world, is forbidden. The player violates the spirit of the game. This double function of many constitutive rules is the reason why I suggest that they define what is to be counted as a proper action.

What is to be said about normativity in the medical context? I suggested that, for instance, rehabilitation personnel have to fixate their language in order to communicate properly. One way of doing this is to specify activities such as walking, talking, and reading in terms of acts (walking 50 yards) or in terms of characteristics such as speed and balance in the performance of the activity. Such things could be standardized and itemized in classificatory lists. This is partly done in the *ICIDH (The International Classification of Impairments, Disabilities and Handicaps)*. Is this at all different than the standardization used in science? Is it not just the case that the health care personnel create their own technical language?

To a great extent this is the case. Owing to the different purposes in the different practices, differences in emphasis may exist. In health care an emphasis exists on the minimal standard for proper action. The person who cannot walk, talk, or read properly has not fulfilled the minimal standard for walking, talking, or reading which has been set up as the goal of rehabilitation. The question then is: minimal for what? The answer is that the purposes can vary somewhat. If a person cannot perform properly according to such a standard then he or she may be entitled to care or further rehabilitation.

Quite a different kind of minimal standard exists when people apply to enter a certain sector in life, a school or a profession. A person cannot become an army officer, a sailor, or a police officer unless he or she can perform certain actions properly. In some cases, these lines are not really 'minimal.' Particularly strong requirements exist with regard to certain abilities for the mentioned categories.

Let me conclude about the element of normativity in standards for action.

a. A basic sense of standard exists where 'standard' only refers to the result of a stipulated definition.

b. In legal and administrative definitions of actions, the constitutive standard can also be regulative in the sense that the action in question is obligatory for, or at least expected of, a professional in the relevant sector.

c. In the health care sector a proper action (or rather: the ability to perform a proper action) can be what is desired or required for a certain purpose and be related to a person's right to care and rehabilitation.

1.14.4 Standards of excellence

So far I have been discussing conditions for performing an action at all or performing a minimally proper action. But we can also evaluate actions along a scale of excellence. We can perform an action just in the way required, we can perform it moderately well, we can perform it well, and we can perform it excellently. Some actions can even be quantitatively measured along scales of excellence. This is particularly salient in sports. To run 100 metres in 11 seconds is to run moderately well, to do it in 10.5 is to run very well, and under 10 seconds is excellent. This scale is tuned to real athletes; other scales exist for ordinary people.

Similar evaluations can be made within the fine arts. Artists can perform well along the dimension of aesthetic beauty or other dimensions relevant to the arts: being provocative, being interesting, opening people's minds, etc.

A different kind of evaluation deals with professional excellence. This is quite often, but not universally, a utilitarian evaluation. A person does well in engineering, in plumbing, in health care, etc. if the person promotes the good that the profession has been instituted for. With some professions, such as the scientist's, one is inclined to add that there may be an intrinsic value in performing the professional activity. This holds equally as much for the artist. We often talk about the intellectual value of science that is to be compared to the aesthetic value of art.

What about the moral standards? Do we have a scale of excellence in morals? Certainly we do. A is living a life which has higher moral qualities than B's. But is this evaluation valid also for instances of actions? Can we say that one performance of an action type F is better than another performance of the same action-type from a moral point of view?

This is an interesting question in itself, since the standard moral question is: What action type should be performed in a context like this? For instance: Should one treat an elderly terminally ill person or should one let him or her die? The moral question is often pursued in a dichotomized language: Shall I perform an action of this action-type or of that action-type? Not: What variant of this action-type shall I perform? One reason for this dichotomization of the standard moral talk is that such talk focuses on dramatic situations and it focuses on what is one's duty and on what is plainly morally wrong. The moral philosopher rarely faces questions concerning degrees of moral excellence. But perhaps it could be worthwhile doing so and considering parallels with other kinds of excellence. Could we then say that a certain action can be performed in a morally better way than it is normally done? And how should this locution be analysed? Here we seem to be forced to consider the question of individuation of action-types.

The most inclusive actions conceivable, such as living one's life, can be performed more or less well from a moral point of view. Similar is the case with slightly less, but still considerably, inclusive actions, such as living one's professional life, leading one's personnel, etc. It is natural to explain why it sounds all right to claim that A is living his life in a morally better way than B by considering the quantity of good actions or bad actions (embedded in the higher-level actions) performed by the agents in question. But what when we consider a specific level? What about the possibility of giving a gift in a more or less moral way? What about telling about the death of a person to a relative of this person in a more or less moral way?

Consider the following. If you give your mother a gift in a very indifferent way not showing any affection, you do not make her very happy. You can even be said to violate her right to your affection. If you tell a father that his son has died in a car accident in a very brusque way then this is very obviously an act with a lower moral value than if you do it carefully and with respect. This type of case has a prominent place in medical ethics. Communication is a field in medical ethics where the way you say things is equally important as what you say.

A critic can say that the how-questions here are arbitrary. You can always create act-categories such as distinguish the morally appropriate ones from the morally improper ones. The morally good ways to communicate then constitute one set of action-types, and the morally worse ways constitute another set of action-types. Thus we can eliminate the talk about ways of performing altogether. An answer to this, though, is that this move of elimination can be artificially pursued for all scales of excellence. The athletically, artistically, and scientifically excellent actions can form a special set of action-types and can thus be separated from the less excellent ones. Such a procedure, however, is hardly suitable for practical purposes. If a clear scale exists along which a person can move in training and rehabilitation, then it is important to see the scale and the progress. The process of development can be concealed by using different act-categories. Similarly, a person can practise communicating in a way that fulfils moral standards better. Such differences may be detected if we consider different degrees of sensitivity and different degrees of care. My conclusion therefore is that the idea of differentiating degrees of excellence can, and should, be used also in the case of moral excellence.

1.15 **Summary concerning classification of actions**

Above, I have made a number of distinctions among actions. These distinctions are of very different order. First, I have made the fundamental logical distinction between action-types and action-instances, and between action-types of various degrees of specification. Second, I have distinguished between such actions as have a terminating end, the acts, and such as do not, the activities. Third, I have noted that actions may be distinguished along dimensions of complication. I have focused on two such dimensions. One dimension concerns the number of conditions in the external world that have to be fulfilled in order for an action of a certain type to occur. This led me to the fundamental distinction between natural actions and conventional actions, the latter being actions which have come into being through conventional stipulation. The second dimension concerns how actions can be added to each other to form action-complexes, by me called action-chains and action-sequences. Furthermore I have distinguished between rational and irrational actions in different senses of these terms. Finally, I have discussed and tried to assess the appropriateness of the idea of degrees of excellence with regard to actions. These grounds for divisions among actions are certainly not the only conceivable ones.

We can conceive of other forms of complexity, for instance the degree of effort needed for performing the basic action(s) involved. We can classify basic actions as to anatomical location. We can classify actions as to their significance and place in human life. These are kinds of classification that are pertinent to the field of health care and to which I will return in Part 2 of this book.

Chapter 2

On the possibilities for action: ability, opportunity, authority, and competence

2.1 Introduction

My analysis of actions has already pointed to the multitude of conditions that have to exist for an action to be realized. Apart from a bodily movement, a mental action, or an omission, there are many aspects of the external world that must be in order. The external world must provide the *opportunity* for the action to take place. And for the necessary bodily movement or mental action to occur, the person must have the *ability* to perform it. For some conventional actions, a further requirement exists. In order to perform certain institutional acts the agent must also be endowed with an *authority*. Only an authorized judge can sentence a criminal; and only a priest (or equivalent person) can marry a couple. The 'can' here does not mean 'is allowed to'. It is a substantial 'can' in the sense that unauthorized persons will not succeed in creating the desired results. The criminal will not be sentenced and the couple will not become married if unauthorized persons attempt to perform the actions in question.

When a person has both ability, opportunity, and in special cases authority to perform *F*, then we shall say that there is a *practical possibility* for this person to perform *F*. Practical possibility is the strongest form of ability. If *A* has the practical possibility for performing *F* and tries to perform *F*, then *A* performs *F*. Trying could then be used as a test for practical possibility.

Let me, in the following, focus on the notions of ability and opportunity and their interrelations. Abilities and opportunities are concepts that indicate *dimensions*. One can have more or less of an ability, and an opportunity can be more or less adequate. John can be a good driver and a bad driver, meaning that he has more or less of the ability to drive. A particular tennis court may provide a good opportunity to play tennis this year; last year, however, it was in a poor condition and provided a bad opportunity.

Ability and opportunity are concepts that are logically interrelated in the following strong sense: When *A* is said to be able to perform *F*, then this is so, given a particular set of circumstances C. John may be able to row a boat when the sea is calm. He is unable to do so, however, when it is stormy. And, conversely, when A is said to have an opportunity to perform F, then this is so, given a particular internal setup I. The tennis court provides an opportunity to play tennis for Sara, now that she is well trained. Last year, however, when she knew nothing about tennis, the court would not give her any opportunity to play.

Thus, there is no such thing as ability *per se*. And there is no such thing as an opportunity *per se*. A person's ability must be judged in the light of a certain set of circumstances. And a person's opportunity must be judged in the light of a certain set of conditions internal to her body or mind.

But if ability and opportunity are in this way related to each other, what sense can we give to the idea of enabling a person to do something? We say that it is the duty of the health care personnel to try to restore the person's ability to walk or to read. And normally we do not add anything about circumstances. Indeed, most of our ability to talk is conducted in absolute terms. We say about our fellow human beings that they can walk, drive cars, speak certain languages, etc. Strictly speaking, this must be elliptic talk. There cannot be any absolute abilities of these kinds. So what do we mean when we ascribe *abilities simpliciter* to people?

We can discern two important interpretations of this mode of speech. They are not rival candidates. I think it is clear that in some cases one interpretation is the true one. In other cases the other interpretation is probably correct. According to the first interpretation, a person is said to have ability, given that *standard circumstances* obtain. According to the second interpretation, he or she is said to have this ability, given that *reasonable circumstances* obtain. Let me comment on both alternatives.

In most cases when I claim that John is able to walk, I mean that this is so, given that there is nothing unusual that would prevent the execution of his action. The weather should not be extremely bad, the ground should not be extremely rough, and there should be no direct obstacles preventing him from walking. Given the way the world normally is – and in particular the way John's immediate surroundings normally are – John is able to walk.

Situations occur when the idea of standard circumstances fails to account for our way of talking about ability. Consider the following case of a school teacher in Chechenya. He has been well trained for his profession, he has a good talent for teaching and we would certainly describe him as a good teacher, i.e. able to teach young pupils. However, Chechenya is a country that has for a long time been deprived of most reasonable opportunities. Most schools have been closed and there have been few if any possibilities of providing regular teaching. This has also meant that our school teacher has not been able to teach.

This situation of deprivation has for some time been the standard situation in Chechenya. Hence, the school teacher is unable, given standard circumstances, to teach. This is a strict application of the first interpretation. But surely, we would say that he is capable of teaching. We must then have made a different presupposition. For instance, we might mean that he is able to teach, given *reasonable* circumstances. In a reasonable world, where institutions are well organised the teacher in question would be able to teach.

However, the school teacher could be judged as being able to teach also given a slightly different interpretation of the notion of standard circumstances. The term 'standard' need not be limited to a particular time and a particular region. If 'standard' is taken to refer to the global community, then the school teacher must be said to be able to teach. He would succeed in teaching in most other countries. The situation in Chechenya is non-standard from a global point of view. This may be so in this particular case. The distinction between standard and reasonable may nevertheless be important. There could be several contexts where we would call a particular circumstance reasonable while it is clearly not the statistically most common circumstance from a global point of view. For instance, much technological equipment exists which is standard in the prosperous world. We who live there take this standard for granted and judge the abilities of our fellow human beings from this point of view. Most of us in the rich world would fail to manage life without this equipment. We would be unable to live given the statistically most common circumstances. We are able to live, however, given the reasonable circumstances (in the rich world).

2.2 Conditions of success

The analysis of such factors as are needed for the success of actions can be made in a more detailed way than the notions of ability, opportunity, authority, and competence allow. Moreover, given our classification of actions into simple and more complex ones, we can look at the differences between the numbers and types of factors needed for the various kinds of actions. In this section I will pursue this analysis in a more systematic way.

Consider now the conditions for a person's practical possibility of acting. These conditions differ, of course, depending on the type of action and on whether we are talking about ability or opportunity. I shall first discuss conditions for *ability*, and such conditions will hold for all kinds of action, in particular for *basic actions*.

I will first take into account the fact that actions are intended. A general ability to perform an action thus presupposes an ability to form the intention to perform the action in question. This indicates that certain mental preparation is necessary for a person to act. It is impossible for A to intend to perform F if

A is completely unaware of *F*. This kind of situation is not so common with basic actions as with many generated actions. (See the discussion below.) Still, the point is also relevant for basic actions. People are not aware of all the possible movements they can make with their limbs. Hence, there are certain movements they will never intend to make.

Also, there are mental factors that may prevent a person from performing a particular action. The person may find an action so revolting that he or she would never intend to perform it. This again is more common with certain complex actions; most unethical actions, for instance, are complex actions. A further interesting case of mental prevention is the one where an agent is continually convinced that he or she is not physically able to perform the action in question. If this is so the agent will never form the intention to perform it.

Thus, factors such as ignorance about an action, revulsion against it, or conviction of one's physical inability, will prevent the realization of the first stage in acting, intending to act and setting about acting. These factors, which are not generally acknowledged in the context of ability, have particular importance for the theory of health. Many types of mental diseases can be located in defects among the antecedents of intending.

For the realization of the second stage of action, its actual performance and success, there are certain obvious requirements. With basic actions these requirements all concern the biological make-up of the agent. This make-up can be divided into various aspects. One is that the agent must not be paralyzed. Other aspects involve such things at that the muscle tissues be sufficiently developed, the joints function properly, and so on.

The condition of opportunity is easy to characterize in the case of basic actions. Here opportunity consists merely in the non-existence of external preventive factors. A man has the opportunity to raise his hand if nothing physically prevents his doing so.

These, then, are the background conditions for the practical possibility of performing a basic action. Consider now the complex actions *accomplishments* and *projects*. By definition, the performance of an accomplishment requires the performance of some basic action. A second requirement is that the accomplishment can *in fact* be generated, i.e. that the generating mechanism is in order. A third requirement is that the agent knows that there is a situation that constitutes the opportunity to generate the accomplishment in question. This entails either that the person has some causal knowledge, i.e. knows what happens, given a particular basic action in a particular situation, or that he or she has some conventional knowledge, i.e. knows of a particular action-generating rule and what it says about the required circumstances. (In some cases both kinds of knowledge may be presupposed.)

I will now collect these requirements (together with the ones noted above) into one schema. The following symbols will be used: *Acc* for accomplishment, *Pro* for project, *B* for basic action, *O* for opportunity, and *S* for action-sequence.

It is practically possible for *A* to perform an accomplishment *Acc* if, and only if,

(i) there is an action-chain, *B* … *Acc*, given an opportunity *O*;

(ii) *A* believes that (i), feels no revulsion against performing *Acc*, and believes that he or she is physically able, given the circumstances, to perform *Acc*;

(iii) it is practically possible for *A* to perform *B*;

(iv) *O* is present;

(v) *A* identifies *O*.

I will now turn to the case of projects. The practical possibility of carrying out a project must involve the practical possibility of performing each action that is a member of some action-sequence constituting the project. (As I have said, there are often alternative ways of carrying out the project.) But the practical possibility of performing each member of a set of accomplishments does not suffice for the performance of the project. Again the agent must have a considerable amount of knowledge. I can summarize the items that he or she must know:

(i) *A* must be aware of at least one action-sequence constituting the project.

(ii) *A* must know what constitutes the opportunity for all members of this sequence.

(iii) *A* must know how these opportunities are to be identified.

A further important element in the performance of some projects is the element of *coordination*. It is sometimes required that one cannot only perform each of the basic actions or accomplishments involved in the project, but also coordinate them into a sequence with special properties (for instance, properties of time, force or elegance). For instance, to produce a melody it is clearly not enough to produce the right notes, one at a time. The components of the melody must be coordinated in a particular way for the result to be music.

I will express the requirements for carrying out a project in the proposed formal manner:

It is practically possible for *A* to carry out the project *Pro* if, and only if,

(i) there is an action-sequence *S*: *Acc*1 … *Accn* constituting *Pro*;

(ii) *A* believes that (i), feels no revulsion against carrying out *Pro* and believes that he or she is physically able, given the circumstances, to perform *Pro*;

(iii) it is practically possible for A to perform each of $Acc1 \ldots Accn$, given their respective opportunities;

(iv) A is able to coordinate each of $Acc1 \ldots Accn$ in the appropriate way;

(v) the required opportunities actually arise;
and

(vi) A identifies these opportunities.

2.3 On not being able to act

My analysis of the notion of practical possibility for action provides us with the tools for seeing the variety of reasons why people are sometimes not able to perform the actions they want to perform. I shall sum up below the nature of such factors as can prevent the realization of an action. I shall thereby use the concepts and the distinctions previously introduced in this book.

Non-ability to perform a basic action, say the movement of one's leg, can be due to a neurophysiological disorder, immediate external prevention or a serious mental disorder, entailing weakness of will. This, then, is a rather limited set of factors.

Non-ability to perform an accomplishment Acc can be seen to depend on not less than the following factors:

(i) No action-chain $X \ldots Acc$ exists, where X is a variable for basic actions;

(ii) A is not aware of any action-chain $X \ldots Acc$;

On the supposition that there is an action-chain $B \ldots Acc$ known to A, we have the following possibilities:

(iii) A is not able to perform B;

(iv) A does not know about his or her ability to perform B;

(v) No opportunity for Acc by the performance of B exists;

(vi) A does not identify any opportunity for Acc.

Let me illustrate some of these reasons for non-ability by considering the accomplishment of starting the engine of a car. A may be unable to start the car for the reason that

(i) The engine has broken down. There is no mechanism being initiated by the starting button;

(ii) A does not know of any way of starting the engine;

(iii) A has broken his or her right hand and cannot press the starting button;

(iv) A does not know that he or she can move the hand properly. (He or she is, for instance, not aware that the hand has healed after having been broken);

(v) *A* is not in the right position to press the button. He or she may be at some other place and hence there is no opportunity for starting the car;

(vi) Although *A* is in the right position in the car he or she cannot find the button.

In accordance with this schema it is then easy to see how non-ability to perform a project will be analysed.

2.4 **On dependencies between abilities**

Just as actions are linked to one another in chains and sequences, so too are abilities. If John is able to cut wood by using a motor saw, but not by any other means, then one can say that his ability to cut wood is dependent on his ability to use a motor saw. There are a few observations to make about abilities and their interrelatedness that are important for my further task. In the example I just gave there was an *individual* dependence. John's ability to cut wood was dependent on his ability to use a motorsaw. Likewise Sara's ability to write a dissertation in English is dependent on her mastery of the English language. But there are also *general* dependencies, wherein the individual agent is without relevance. If there is only one existing procedure to realize a certain state – if *G-ing* is the only existing way to *F* – then there is a general dependency between the ability to *F* and the ability to *G*. This is quite often the case when it comes to conventional actions and conventional abilities. By a convention one can always stipulate that there should be just one procedure by which, for instance, a governmental bill can be issued.

In line with my further observations concerning action generation we can discern different kinds of dependencies, in particular *causal* and *conventional* dependencies. An interesting question is whether there are also conceptual dependencies in the area of ability. This question is of particular interest in the field of mental ability. But let me here say a few words about the general idea of conceptual dependency.

The general idea is the following. Assume that we identify a particular ability as the ability to *F*. Assume also that the accepted definition of *F* entails that the agent of *F-ing* must also be *G-ing*. Then the ability to *F* conceptually depends on the ability to *G*. Let me illustrate. Reading a book conceptually entails looking at a page of the book (one cannot read for conceptual reasons without looking at a text), kicking a ball conceptually entails moving one's leg, laughing conceptually entails moving one's facial muscles, etc.

An important distinction exists between these conceptual dependencies and conventional stipulations. No conventional rules have been laid down at a particular time which have created the actions of reading, kicking, or laughing, in the way acts of marrying and sentencing criminals have been created within frameworks of institutions. Reading, kicking, and laughing are natural action verbs, which have certain connotations given in the common language. These connotations may be codified in dictionaries. But the definitions found in dictionaries are not like conventional stipulations, they just notify a linguistic practice that already exists.

I am aware that we can find difficult borderline cases here. We may wonder what is to be required of a conventional rule. We may wonder whether it must have been written down, etc. There may be conventional actions created a very long time ago, and where we are not aware of this fact. We take the action now as identifiable in the natural action language.

Even granted this fact I think that we need a distinction between conventional actions and natural actions. At any particular time a clear difference exists between such actions as just 'exist' and which we cannot do anything about, and such actions as can be created and changed by fiat. At any time an authority can change, by decision, the conditions and criteria of a conventional action. One can change the rules of marrying and sentencing criminals. One can at a particular time loosen the requirements for marrying. One can abolish the requirement concerning witnesses, for instance, or one can let all legally competent adults act as marriage officials. Or, more radically, one can abolish the concept of marriage altogether. One may replace it by something different – a partnership relation – for instance, which has new and different legal implications.

My conclusion then is: at any time we can fairly well identify a set of natural actions and a set of conventionally created and conventionally defined actions. Among the natural actions we can find certain pairs that stand in a conceptual relationship to one another. An interesting question now is: can we also talk about *conceptual generation* of actions, as we have talked about causal and conventional generation? I think it is in principle possible. But the question is if there is any need. One can consider the relation of all the cases above as causal. Looking at a text causally contributes to reading. Moving one's leg causally contributes to kicking, etc. We here have a causal relation covered by one and the same concept.

2.5 On first- and second-order abilities

We may talk of ability of different orders. I will here distinguish between first- and second-order ability. So far, both my discussion and my characterizations have concerned first-order ability only. The notion of second-order ability will be defined as follows:

> A has a second-order ability with regard to an action F if, and only if, A has the first-order ability to pursue a training programme after the completion of which A will have the first-order ability to do F.

Second-order *ability* is thus compatible with first-order *disability*, while the reverse does not hold. A may lack the first-order ability to earn her living in Sweden. A may, however, have the second-order ability to do so. A may be able to train to make a good living in that country.

Aristotle (1908) in fact notes the same kind of distinction by introducing the pair *first and second actualizations*. What I here call a second-order ability can be actualized in two steps. First, the second-order ability can, through training, become a first-order ability. This is the first actualization. Then, the first-order ability can be actualized through action. This is the second actualization.

Note that the action of *training* must be given the same analysis as other kinds of action. When we ascribe to someone the first-order ability to follow a particular training programme, we must, as in the general case above, presuppose a set of standard or reasonable circumstances. We must moreover presuppose that it persists throughout the training process. Thus, a person who enters on a training programme, but in the end fails to acquire the desired first-order ability, need not lack second-order ability. First, the training programme may have been poor. This might indicate that the accepted circumstances did not obtain. Second, the subject may, after a while, no longer have intended to pursue the training in a proper way. This being so is still consistent with his or her having the second-order ability. Second-order ability may not turn into first-order ability if the agent does not consistently try to acquire the first-order ability.

Consider now the following case. Some subjects are afforded adequate training facilities, and they try to learn through the whole period designated for training. Nevertheless, after this period they still do not know how to perform the desired action. This indicates that the subjects do not have the second-order ability, at least not through the whole period of training, to perform the action. We could then say that they are *genuinely disabled* with respect to performing the action in question.

To summarize: Persons have a second-order disability with regard to an action *F* if, and only if, they are disabled, given standard or reasonable circumstances, with regard to consistently pursuing a training programme to acquire a first-order ability to perform *F*.

The notion of second-order ability brings us closer to the biologically founded capabilities of human beings. Nevertheless, it does not and cannot completely free us from the relativity of an action to an environment. To say that A has a first-order ability to follow a training programme successfully presupposes, as I have said, a particular set of circumstances. It may be conceivable that certain people who lack a first-order ability could, if they were put into extremely advanced and extremely expensive training programmes, achieve the first-order ability desired. But if such programmes have not been offered, or if they have not even been designed, they cannot be taken into account in ascribing second-order ability to people.

These observations have a great impact in an analysis of the medical notion of disability and handicap, as well as in the analysis of health (see Chapter 3).

2.6 **On different levels of ability**

Above I have attempted to analyse in some detail the components of the locution 'ability to perform an intentional action'. I will now argue that this analysis is not quite adequate as an analysis of all our language with regard to ability. We may easily find examples where it is true to say that A is able to do F, and A has the opportunity to do F, but A would still not perform F even if A were to try. Consider the following cases:

A can count to one billion, but if she tries today she will probably not succeed because she is so tired that she will fall asleep after having counted to a couple of thousand.

A can issue a licentiate's degree, but this term A is on sabbatical leave so at the moment she is not entitled to do so.

A can write a book on the nature of health, but she is at present not feeling well, so there is little chance that this book will materialize this year.

A can play football but she has broken her leg so she won't play any football this month.

What then is the point of saying that one *is able* to do all these things? What is the information conveyed and in what way is this information related to the counterfactual: if A were to try to do F, then A would do F?

Part of the analysis here is commonplace. The counterfactual constitutes the analysis of a very strong notion of 'can', namely the notion of *practical possibility*. This notion refers to the situation when all necessary conditions – which together with trying are sufficient for a particular action – are materialized. When it is practically possible for me to do F, then it is true of me that, if I were to try to do F, then I would do F. Ability, as I have said, constitutes the person's internal conditions for performing an action, opportunity of external conditions for performing the same action. In certain cases there is also some legal authority required. One of my examples involves the latter factor of authority. The issuing of a licentiate's degree fails because of lack of authority. The agent is on sabbatical leave.

But what is missing in the other cases? Can one say that A has the ability but not the opportunity to count, or that A has the ability but not the opportunity to write the book or play football? This does not seem right given the preliminary characterization of opportunity as an external circumstance that enables a person to succeed in a particular task. Nothing exists which externally prevents the person from counting. Likewise, no external impediments exist for the writer or the footballer.

More layers and degrees of possibility of action exist which cannot simply be accounted for by the distinctions between ability, opportunity, and authority. My next task is to investigate these.

2.7 The distinction between a physical and a mental aspect of ability

My task now is to answer the following question: How could we justify saying that the person who is to count, the potential author, and the footballer are able to perform their respective actions, and where are we to find the elements lacking for the successful performance of their tasks? I have suggested that ability is multilayered. An agent may fulfil the ability conditions in some of these layers but fail in respect of others. But which are the principal layers? Do some fundamentally different senses of 'ability' exist which play a part in this context?

In this section I will test the hypothesis that a distinction exists between a person's physical and mental ability to perform an action. A person may be able to do something in a mental sense but not in a physical sense. My hypothesis then is: the ability ascribed to the persons in our three examples is some kind of mental ability. They lack, however, the relevant physical ability for succeeding in their tasks. In testing this hypothesis I will briefly investigate the mental conditions for the ability of performing a physical action. In this process I will argue that all abilities to perform a physical action have certain mental conditions.

I will turn to the latter issue first. I think all actions, at least all action-types, have a mental ingredient. This follows, I believe, from the fact, first, that actions are per definition intentional, and, second, that intending to do F entails believing that it is practically possible to do F. A man cannot intend to travel to Brazil unless he believes that it is practically possible for him to make this journey. He may wish to do so, without the relevant belief, but intending is a much stronger species of will. (See my analysis of decisions and intentions in Chapter 1, Section 1.3.)

Thus, if A is able to perform the intentional action F, then A must be able to form the relevant belief concerning her possibility of performing F. This holds for the simplest of actions, for instance the basic action of raising one's arm. An ability to form a belief is thus an element of all ability to be discussed here.

This is not the whole story. An ability to perform a physical action presupposes some minimal perception and some bodily consciousness. The agent must have some perception of the environment and must know where she has her arm in order to direct her energy in the right direction. A further requirement is the ability to *identify* the opportunity for the action in question. All action, even the most basic, presupposes, as I have said, an opportunity. The raising of one's arm presupposes that there are no impediments, nothing that actually prevents the movement of the arm. The persons who set themselves to raise their arms must therefore identify the presence of the right opportunity.

Thus, ability to perform a physical action entails the existence of a mental faculty in the sense that the agent must be able to form beliefs and that he or she must be a perceiving individual with a sophisticated bodily consciousness. If we leave the basic actions and turn to generated actions, the picture, as we have seen, becomes even more salient. The agent must know the generating mechanism and must identify the right opportunities for all the subactions constituting the chain.

I will now turn back to my initial question and my examples: Is it true to say that the person who counts, the author, and the footballer have the relevant mental ability for performing their respective actions but lack the relevant physical ability? (For a full account of mental ability, see Chapter 3, Section 3.2.) The person who counts knows indeed the generating mechanism involved in counting, she knows how to generate a new number after having said a certain number; but in my example the person does not have the physical strength to continue after a while. Likewise, the author knows in principle what to do in order to write the relevant book, but she is not well and therefore lacks the necessary energy. Similarly, the footballer knows how to play, but is impeded from playing by a broken leg.

As far as my observations go, they seem to be correct. It is doubtful, however, to claim that the crucial distinction should be between the physical and the mental. Some mental elements exist which need not be relevant to the sense of ability that I am seeking, and, as I will shortly argue, some physical elements exist which are relevant.

Consider first some irrelevant mental ingredients. It is questionable whether fatigue is just physical. We often talk about mental fatigue. And the feeling of fatigue clearly is a mental property. The woman who counts may very well stop counting because she feels tired. Still, we say that she can count to a billion. A certain mental inability is compatible with the person's ability in the sense we are trying to determine here. Moreover, both the woman who counts, the author, and the footballer may be inattentive when they try to perform their actions. They may fail to identify opportunities in their enterprises and thereby not succeed in completing their actions. Such mental inability, at least when it is understood as temporary, is compatible with the ability that I am seeking to identify.

Moreover, people may, through illness, temporarily have lost their bodily consciousness and their capacity to identify relevant opportunities, but they may still have the ability in question. The relevant condition for ascribing the ability I am seeking must have to do, then, with some more specific mental property. A plausible hypothesis is that it has to do with the person's knowledge, in particular with what is often called his or her *know-how*.

2.8 **On ability, know-how, and competence**

The woman who can count to a billion knows how to count; she knows all the rules concerning how to generate any number in the series of natural numbers. The author in our example similarly knows how to write a scientific book; she knows all the conventions and rules for producing a text acceptable to a scientific publisher. Similarly, the footballer knows the rules of football and knows how to outplay the members of the opposing team. Knowledge is clearly a crucial element in the ability that we ascribe to the three agents under discussion. Less clear is that this knowledge has to be theoretical. Furthermore, it is quite doubtful that knowledge is all that is at issue.

Ever since Gilbert Ryle's famous essay 'Knowing How and Knowing That' (1971) it is commonplace to distinguish between theoretical knowledge, i.e. knowledge-that, and practical knowledge, i.e. knowledge-how. In having a piece of theoretical knowledge one knows that a set of propositions is true. In having a piece of practical knowledge one knows how to perform an action or how to reach a goal. This distinction is fruitful but not entirely clear. A fully satisfactory application of it requires a number of further clarifications. Since my presentation does not rely on the distinction I confine myself to the following remarks. Knowing-that and knowing-how, however further clarified, must be related to each other. In some cases knowing that X may even be sufficient for knowing how to do F, and in many cases knowing that X is necessary for knowing how to do F. Among my three examples the relation between knowing-that and knowing-how is perhaps strongest in the case of the arithmetician. This person's knowledge of a set of mathematical truths may be sufficient for her know-how. In the case of the author there is still a strong relation, but it seems quite plausible that some of the author's know-how cannot be translated into true propositions. In the case of the footballer most of her knowledge is of the practical kind and not translatable into theoretical knowledge.

But is knowledge, whether of the theoretical or the practical kind, ever sufficient for saying that the agent is able to perform a particular action? In answering this question, I will start with the footballer, where the grounds for doubt are the strongest. Are we inclined to say that A can play football simply on the ground that she knows how to play football? Consider a former footballer, a 75-year-old man, who has ever since his active years worked as a radio commentator on football and has supreme knowledge, both theoretical and practical, about the game. In a perfectly understandable sense, this person knows how to play football. But clearly this man no longer has the ability to play football, in the sense we are seeking. He has, as we say, lost the relevant *skill*. He is no longer well trained; he cannot move quickly enough, he does not react quickly enough and he no longer has the required physical strength.

I will at this stage introduce what I take to be a crucial concept for my analytical task, namely the concept of *competence*. The competent footballer has both know-how and skill. In many areas of activity, perhaps ultimately in all areas, there is a combination of know-how and skill required for complete competence. This holds very clearly for painters, musicians, and people who do handicraft. All these people need a skill to modulate and coordinate bodily movements that goes far beyond any kind of knowledge. But the same probably holds true to some extent for all enterprises.

To let the notion of skill also enter the mental field is crucial. In fact the distinction between the mind and the body is hard to uphold here. In the case of painters and musicians, similarly with athletes and circus artists, their training is as much a training of the mind as a training of the body. Their skill comprises not only a trained body, that has strength, plasticity, and is capable of rapid movement, but comprises also a capacity for identifying more and more subtle nuances, whether it be in one's body, in one's task or in one's environment.

Let me summarize. I have identified an important notion of competence, constituted by know-how and by physical and mental skill. Supported by my examples I argue that the term 'ability' and its verbal associate 'being able' sometimes refer to competence and not to full ability. The person who counts has the competence for counting to a billion, but since he or she soon gets sick and tired of counting, does not succeed in doing so. The author and the footballer likewise have the competence for their respective tasks, but fail to realize them because of lack of attention, fatigue or injury.

Typical is that competence is a more enduring and basic state of the human being than full ability is. For temporary reasons, such as the ones mentioned above, the person may be prevented from execution of this competence. But when we look upon the situation precisely in these terms, i.e. as a situation of prevention from the execution of a competence, we say that the competence is still there. This statement is compatible with the recognition of the fact that also competence may get lost. Cases of illness exist which permanently or for a long time destroy some basic properties of the person, including his or her competence to perform many tasks.

To say, then, that a person can perform F, in the competence sense of can, is tantamount to saying something general and basic about this person. It belongs to the same level of abstraction as describing the personality of the person. We say of a particular man that he is of the *kind* that can do such and such. But saying that a man is of such a kind does not entail that he will at any moment, when he tries and where the right opportunity is there, succeed in doing such and such. The general competence is distinct from present full ability.

Chapter 3

Towards a theory of health and illness

3.1 Health as ability to realize vital goals

3.1.1 Introduction

There is an ongoing controversy concerning the nature of health and illness in many health-related disciplines. Two mainstreams have appeared in the arena. One of them is medical or biological. What is typical of protagonists of this stream of thought is that they claim that the concepts of health and illness can be treated as purely biological concepts. 'Health' and 'illness' are taken to be biological concepts in the same sense as 'heart' and 'blood pressure' are biological concepts. There is nothing, it is claimed, subjective or evaluative about these concepts. I shall call this the *naturalist* line of thought.

The other mainstream involves a completely opposite position with regard to these matters. According to the *holists*, health and illness are concepts pertaining to the whole person in his or her social context. In their view, health concepts must be formulated in psycho-social or even sociological terms. Thus, a biological or psychological characterization is not enough. To say that somebody is healthy partly means that this person can function in his or her social context.

My own position is on the holistic side (1995; 2001). I have argued extensively against naturalism, in particular against its most celebrated version presented by the American philosopher Christopher Boorse (1977; 1997). This theory is based on the general idea that being healthy is natural in the sense of being biologically normal. According to Boorse's explication, biological (or medical) functional normality is relative to the goals 'physiologists seem to assume, viz. individual survival and reproduction' (1997, p. 9). This functional normality is to be determined by statistical means.

I will confine myself here to presenting one basic argument in favour of a holistic view as against a bio-statistical conception. This is an argument based on the so-called reverse theory of disease and illness. (The term was coined by Fulford 1989, but essentially the same thought exists in Canguilhem 1978; see also Nordenfelt's (2001) expansion of the argument.) Consider the following, hopefully plausible, story with regard to the emergence of the concepts of illness and disease. This story is essentially a (shortened) paraphrase of Fulford's explication of the priority relations between the concepts of dysfunction, illness, and disease.

1. In the beginning, there were people who experienced problems in and with themselves. They felt pain and fatigue, and they found themselves unable to do what they could normally do. They experienced what we now call illnesses, which they located somewhere in their bodies and minds. Many people came to experience similar illnesses. This led to the giving of names to the illnesses, and hereby the presence of the illnesses could be efficiently communicated. These were the phases of *illness recognition* and *illness communication*.

2. The ill people approached experts, called doctors, in order to get help. They communicated their experiences to the doctors, via the illness language. The doctors tried to help them and cure them. In the search for curative remedies, the doctors did not just rely on the stories told by the ill people. They also looked for the *causes* of the illnesses within the bodies and minds of the ill. This meant in the end that they initiated systematic studies of the biology of their patients. This was the phase of *search for the causes of illnesses*.

As a result of these studies, the doctors found some regular connections between certain bodily states and the illness symptoms of their patients. They formed hypotheses about causal connections between the internal states and processes and the illness syndromes.

3. They designated these causes of illnesses as *diseases*. And they invented a vocabulary and a conceptual apparatus for the diseases. This was the phase of *disease recognition*.

4. Once the diseases were recognized, new and independent research could be established. The diseases as biological processes could be studied in their own right and irrespective of their connection to human suffering. This became the phase of *biomedical research*.

This is a quasi-historical sketch of the development of the notion of disease. According to this story, the concept of illness is primary to the concept of disease. At the heart of the story lies a problem that has to be solved through investigation into the causes of this problem. These causes are assumed to exist within the subject's body or mind.

I find this sketch to be a plausible one also for the explication of the contemporary concepts of illness, disease, and health. Diseases are causes of the problems that we call illnesses. Health is the absence of illnesses. This explication is more plausible than the rival one that says that diseases are bodily states that make a statistically subnormal contribution to the survival and reproduction of their bearers. A problem constituting an illness need not entail a threat to the person's life, growth, or reproduction. The problem quite often concerns pain, other kinds of suffering, or disability. And the subject believes that this problem has some kind of internal (biological or psychological) cause. This is a standard situation where a person is seeking help from a health care institution. I therefore conclude that the concept of disease is related primarily to suffering and disability and not to the probability of death.

3.1.2 Towards a notion of health as ability

Galen (1997) said that health is a state in which we neither suffer from evil nor are prevented from performing the functions of daily life. In a similar vein the American sociologist Talcott Parsons (1972, p. 117) says: 'Health may be defined as the state of optimum capacity of an individual for the effective performance of the roles and tasks for which he has been socialized'.

In such holistic characterizations of health, two kinds of phenomena are often mentioned: first the subjective phenomenon of a certain kind of feeling, of ease or well-being in the case of health, and of pain or suffering in the case of ill health; second the phenomenon of ability or disability, the former an indication of health and the latter of ill health.

These two kinds of phenomena are in many ways interconnected. There is first an empirical, causal, connection. A feeling of ease or well-being contributes causally to the ability of the bearer. A feeling of pain or suffering may directly cause some degree of disability. Conversely, a subject's perception of his or her ability or disability greatly influences his or her emotional state.

Some would argue that the relation between the two kinds of phenomenon is even stronger, i.e. that there are conceptual links between, on the one hand, a feeling of well-being and ability and, on the other hand, suffering and disability. According to this idea, being in great pain, for instance, partly means that one is disabled. Some degree of disability is here a necessary condition for the presence of pain, so that if a person's ability is not affected, the person can be said not to be in great pain.

The assumption of a conceptual relation between pain and disability will be accepted in the present analysis: a person cannot experience great pain or suffering without evincing some degree of disability. But a person may have a disability and even be generally disabled without experiencing pain or suffering. There are some paradigm cases of ill health where pain and suffering are absent. One obvious case is that of coma. Another is certain mental disabilities and illnesses. When a patient cannot reflect on his or her own situation, then the person's disabilities need not have suffering as a consequence. In short, wherever there is great pain or suffering there is disability, but the converse is not true.

These preliminary observations indicate that the concept of disability has a much more central place in the characterization of ill health than the corresponding concepts of pain and suffering. If only one of these characteristics is essential to the notion of ill health, then disability is the primary candidate. This is my main reason for founding the subsequent analysis on the concepts of ability and disability.

3.1.3 The ability of health

What should a healthy person be able to do? Or, conversely, what kinds of disabilities constitute a reduction of the person's health? What disabilities are such that the health care system should provide health care for the person? These questions are clearly not identical. The last question has a political overtone. The answer to it depends not only on conceptual analysis but equally on policy decisions concerning medical priorities. I shall not enter into a discussion of this here.

It is plausible to believe that whatever the adequate answer to the question of the nature of health should be, it will be an answer on an abstract level, which can be summarized in terms of certain general goals. The question to be put should then rather be formulated in the following terms: what are the goals that a healthy person must be able to realize through his or her actions?

My general proposal is the following: *A is completely healthy if, and only if, A is in a bodily and mental state which is such that A has the second-order ability to realize all his or her vital goals given a set of standard or otherwise reasonable circumstances.* Let me now clarify and to some extent defend this proposal by commenting on the crucial clauses concerning vital goals and second-order ability. I shall be brief with regard to the first clause and instead concentrate on the relation between health and second-order ability. For an analysis of the notions of standard and reasonable circumstances, see Chapter 2, Section 2.1. (Full-length accounts of my conception of health are given in Nordenfelt 1995 and 2001.)

3.1.4 On vital goals

What are the vital goals of a human being? And is there just one set of vital goals? A vital goal of a person, I suggest, is a state of affairs that is necessary for this person's minimal long-term happiness. As a consequence of this interpretation many of the things that human beings hope to realize or maintain belong to their vital goals. More precisely, most states which have a high priority along a person's scale of preferences belong to his or her vital goals. Examples of such vital goals can be passing an exam, getting married and having children, as well as simply maintaining elements in the *status quo* such as retaining one's job and remaining in touch with one's nearest and dearest.

However, certain things that people happen to want do not belong to their vital goals. First we have trivial wants. People may casually want something, but if they don't get it, it does not matter much. Second, people may sometimes have counterproductive wants. They may want to get drunk, but getting drunk is not a vital goal. Instead of contributing to long-term happiness, being drunk contributes in the long run to suffering and thereby unhappiness. Third, we may have irrational wants, i.e. wants that are in conflict with other, more important wants. As soon as the agent realizes this conflict, he or she normally realizes that the only candidates for vital goals are the more important wants. (For complications in this picture, see Chapter 6, Section 6.4, on irrational wants.)

On the other hand, some things that we do not want may be contained in our set of vital goals. The completely apathetic or lazy person who does not have any conscious goals whatsoever will soon realize that this creates suffering for him or her. This will be particularly salient if the person does not even seek food or shelter. It must certainly belong to this person's long-term minimal happiness to have these basic matters organized. Therefore, such basic goals are among every person's vital goals.

A crucial observation to be made here, then, is that a vital goal of *A* need not be wanted by *A* at a particular moment. The notion of a vital goal is thus a technical notion partially distinct from the ordinary-language notion of a goal.

3.1.5 On health and second-order ability

Let me here defend the idea of founding the notion of health and second-order ability. To be healthy, I said, is to have the second-order ability to realize one's vital goals. Consider the following situation. A refugee from, say, an African country, has just moved to Sweden. In his native country he had his own business, which he managed well enough to sustain himself and his family. When he enters Sweden he is no longer able to lead such a life. He does not know Swedish culture and, in particular, the Swedish language so he cannot initially make any arrangements for establishing a business in Sweden. Whereas in his home country he lived relatively well, in Sweden he is disabled. But would we say that this man is healthy in his native country, and becomes ill upon entering Sweden? No, it seems more plausible to say that as long as he has the second-order ability to run a business in Sweden, then he remains healthy. This means: as long as the immigrant has the ability to learn the Swedish language and the ability to learn how to go about in our society, then he is a completely healthy person.

In general, then, disability that is solely due to lack of training is not an indication of ill health. There is reason to speak of ill health only if training has in turn been prevented by internal factors, in which case there is a second-order disability.

But what about the typical case of ill health that is due to an organic disease? Consider the following. A woman has a first-order ability to perform her professional activities. Then she becomes ill, and as a result loses her first-order ability. But would it be true to say that she no longer has the second-order ability to do her work?

It is easy to be misled here and identify two pairs of concepts that should be held distinct: one pair is first- and second-order ability, the other is power to execute a basic competence and having a basic competence. We normally ascribe a basic competence to someone when he or she knows how to do something. (See the analysis in Chapter 2, Section 2.8.) According to our previous definition this need not by any means be true of second-order ability. The immigrant to Sweden has not previously learnt anything about Sweden and does not have the basic competence requisite for making his living in Sweden. He may, however, have the second-order ability with regard to the same action.

It is crucial to recognize that a person who has a basic competence vis-à-vis a certain action *F* need not even have a second-order ability with regard to *F*. Consider again the professional footballer who has broken both legs. Obviously, during the ensuing period this person does not have the first-order ability to play football. Still, we would say that the person has throughout the period the basic competence to play football. He or she knows how to play football. But does this person, while lying in bed, have the second-order ability to play football? No, for having the second-order ability to play football means having the first-order ability to follow a training programme that leads to a first-order ability to play football. But the person who is confined to bed is clearly not in a position to follow such a programme; and so we may say of the footballer that he or she is ill.

The same reasoning may be applied to all paradigm cases of ill health due to disease or impairment. During an acute phase of ill health, however short it may be, the subject has lost both the first- and second-order ability to perform the actions with respect to which he or she is disabled.

3.2 On the notions of disease, malady, and illness

So far I have suggested a general characterization of the notion of health. I have also indicated roughly how I find that the notions of disease and illness are related to health. Let me in this section delve more deeply into these notions.

Let me start with 'disease' and treat it together with some other prominent concepts belonging to medicine and pathology, namely 'impairment', 'injury', and 'defect'. Culver and Gert (1982) have collected all these concepts under the common heading of *maladies*. As I see it, maladies have one important feature in common. They are entities internal to the subject's body or mind which tend to compromise his or her health. Thus, for instance, a disease, when occurring in the subject *S*, tends to cause some disability in *S* with respect to one or more of *S*'s vital goals.

I will first comment on the expression 'tends to cause'. The basic idea here is that diseases, although frequently causing ill health, do not always do so. First a disease may be aborted at a very early stage. The disease may be of the kind that it causes disability in its bearer only in the late stages of its development. A similar but not identical reason is that a particular instance of the disease is so mild that its effect on the subject's general ability is negligible.

This preliminary analysis needs to be clarified by the following distinction. On the one hand, a disease can be understood as a *type* of phenomenon; on the other hand it can be understood as an *instance* incorporated in a particular person. The normal labels of diseases, such as 'common cold', 'cancer', and 'tuberculosis', are labels referring to disease types. Tuberculosis is thus a disease type. This type can be instanced in several individuals.

Now my dictum that a disease tends to cause ill health can be understood in two ways: first, most instances of disease-type *D* cause ill health in their bearers; second, disease-instance *I* of *D* will with great probability lead to ill health in its bearer *S*. The second interpretation may be true without the first being true. There may be some properties peculiar to *S* that make *S* particularly vulnerable to *I*.

I have adopted the first interpretation of the general notion of disease as the most reasonable one. I shall say that something is a disease-type *D* only if most instances of it actually compromise health. Something is a disease-instance only if it belongs to a disease type. If we did not have this requirement it would not be possible to have a general science of diseases. Considerations completely analogous to these apply to other maladies, such as impairment, injury, and defect. A presupposition of a general science of maladies is that it deals with types of entities, most instances of which have ill health as a consequence.

But now a crucial question can be asked. How can we establish a universal science of diseases, if in each individual case health is dependent on the person's vital goals? My general answer to this argument is the following. A great many diseases, probably a majority, cause pain, fatigue, and general unease. Such sensations have a tendency to affect *all* kinds of activity. They affect the conditions for performing all basic actions. And since every action requires the performance of some basic action it does not matter very much what the exact vital goals are in a particular population. The diseases would affect most people irrespective of their vital goals.

This general observation does not preclude the existence of *local* diseases for which some local vital goals may be of importance. The paradigm case would be a condition that does not give rise to pain, fatigue, or unease but which only affects a particular ability to reach a particular goal which is deemed vital in a certain cultural context. Consider the following example. A man is – for physiological reasons, and not just because of lack of training – unable to move his ears. Assume that in the culture where he lives the movement of one's ears is an important element of a religious ritual. Taking part in this ritual is a vital goal for this man. In most cultures the ability to move one's ears is entirely irrelevant. This particular talent is almost never practised. Therefore, a local condition pertaining to the ear muscles would almost never be discovered and would not even, I should argue, be deemed a disease or a defect. Here, however, there is a case for speaking of a culture-bound disease dependent on a culture-specific vital goal.

Let me then suggest the following formal characterization of the notion of disease:

> D is a disease type in environment E if, and only if, D is a type of physical or mental process which, when instanced in a person P in E, would with great probability cause ill health in P.

The above concerns the notion of disease which has been chosen as a paradigm notion among the maladies. However, almost everything in the preceding analysis can be seen to be valid also for the other maladies: impairments, injuries, and defects. The essential difference between them has to do with their ontological status. Impairments and defects are mostly taken as being state-like entities, not as being processes, which are continually variable. An injury is either a state or a change of states, i.e. an event. It is an event when one focuses on the moment of incidence, i.e. when the injury as a state comes about. (For the distinction between states, events, and processes, see Nordenfelt, 2000.)

Turn now to the notion of illness. There is some ambivalence in the ordinary use of the term 'illness'. This term is sometimes used to denote the holistic state of ill health, i.e. when health is in general reduced and, in my interpretation, the subject has some disability in relation to his or her vital goals. This is the sense referred to in the locution: *P* is ill. In this book I have chosen the expression 'ill health' to denote this general state of affairs.

There is, however, a more specific use of the term 'illness', i.e. when it refers to a specific pathological condition. In some such contexts 'illness' functions simply as a synonym of 'disease'. In other, more technical discourses, for instance in medical sociology and medical anthropology, 'illness' has a reference distinguishable from that of 'disease'. Roughly, illness is there interpreted as the subjective part of the pathological condition, the suffering and disability, whereas disease is the objective, physiological part of the same condition. I will here propose an explication along such lines. The term 'illness' can be used to combine a number of disabilities into a cluster (or a syndrome). Instead of enumerating each of the disabilities involved in a cluster one can use a common term for the cluster, the illness-term, when this serves scientific or therapeutic purposes. It is particularly convenient to use the illness-term when a cluster is believed to have a common cause, especially when all the disabilities involved in an illness arise from the same disease.

The conceptual suggestion made here provides, in principle, a sharp distinction between illness and disease. Illnesses are typically *effects* of diseases and not identical with them. This scheme has crucial consequences for the field of mental pathology. In fact, most mental 'diseases' would turn out to be illnesses in my terminology. The objects of psychiatric classification are primarily clusters of disabilities, for instance, those with regard to thinking coherently, to communicating, and to socializing. (For further analysis of the disease/illness distinction, see Nordenfelt, 2001, pp. 75–88.)

3.3 On mental actions and mental health

3.3.1 Introduction

In the previous chapter we encountered the ideas of a mental ability and of a mental ingredient in a physical action. I will now go more deeply into the notion of *mental* ability and ask whether it is possible to make a sharp division between mental abilities and physical abilities. This question is interesting and important for many purposes, not least for the theory of health, where a crucial distinction exists between mental and physical health. Moreover, if one sticks to an action-theoretic theory of health, like the one that I have advocated here, it is natural to try to find the key to this distinction in the difference between physical and mental abilities.

But does such a difference exist? One may be tempted to say that all actions, including such actions as involve bodily movements, are mental in the sense that they presuppose the formation of an intention. Intentions, I have been assuming, are mental entities. Clearly, mental capacities may affect all intentional action via the faculty of will. A builder may be perfectly fit physically and from this point of view capable of doing his job, but he may still be unable to do it because of a depression, i.e. an illness that entails a strongly reduced will. Furthermore, as we have seen above, the mental area pervades the physical area in yet further respects. A strong epistemic element is necessary for the performance of all complex physical actions: the agent must know how to perform the action. The action of driving a car is a physical action but it is also a complex action. Clearly, such an action presupposes much knowledge. The agent must not only be minimally physically fit to drive a car; he or she must also know how to drive it. In general, if this knowledge, be it theoretical or practical, is disturbed or even completely removed by illness, the complex action cannot be performed. This strong dependence between physical action and mental ability is, however, asymmetrical. Physical abilities are not necessary for mental actions in the same way.

My reasoning is still very preliminary. I have offered no clear definition of the mental and the physical. For my present purposes, I will here take a short-cut and say that a mental state (or in general a mental episode) is one which does not *logically* entail the existence of any particular physical or bodily state apart from the existence of the bearer of the mental state. To say that a person A understands something does not entail any particular physical state of the universe apart from the physical existence of A. A necessary *empirical* connection may exist between a mental state and a state of the brain, as I have indicated in Chapter 1, Section 1.4, but that is a different story.

This general statement is compatible with the common dispositional analysis of mental *concepts* according to which a mental state entails a disposition to certain physical reactions or actions (Ryle 1949; Armstrong 1968; and Bolton and Hill 2003). To understand something entails capacities or dispositions to act physically in certain ways. When one understands a mathematical formula, one is capable of performing certain technical tasks, involving physical action. However, the mental state and the disposition can exist without such a physical action occurring.

For the analysis of the mental universe I will adopt here a traditional philosophical classification of the mind. According to this classification the mind can be subdivided in terms of so-called *mental faculties*. The exact nature of these faculties, as also the distinction between them, is of course highly debatable. I will not contribute here to this interesting debate. For my purposes it suffices to know that the faculties of cognition (including perception), emotion, and will are among the mental faculties. I will therefore in the following assume that cognitive, emotional, and conative (volitional) abilities are mental abilities.

3.3.2 **Mental ability and mental action**

So much, or so little, about the universe of the mental. But what about a mental *ability*? What is a mental ability related to? In the paradigm use of the general expressions 'A is able to' or 'A is capable of', these expressions are filled out with a locution referring to an intentional action on the part of A. We say that A is able to teach French or A is able to build a house. Here teaching French and building a house are clear examples of intentional actions. Locutions exist, however, where ability can refer to mere dispositions. A child may be able to make a mess of a situation. Here it need not be the case that the child actually intends to do so. The result may be an accident or at least an unintentional result.

The first important question, then, is: do mental intentional actions exist? What can one intend to do where the doing does not involve any physical movements whatsoever? Before concretely considering this question I will make a general observation.

Many mental episodes, although they may be described by verbal locutions that take humans as grammatical subjects, are not actions but instead events or states. (For the concepts of event, state, and process, see Nordenfelt 2000.) A person who understands a problem does not perform any intentional action of understanding. Instead something happens to him or her and remains with him or her for a while, namely as long as the person is in the state of understanding. Likewise a person who hears a sound has normally not intended to hear anything. The hearing of the sound is an event and sometimes remains as a lasting state of the subject. These observations hold true for the emotional and conative faculties as well. No obvious mechanisms by which he or she can intentionally achieve the results of loving, hating, or desiring are available to the ordinary person.

This feature of the mind is typical. The universe of episodes of the mind is much more dominated by states or events, and contains far fewer intentional actions, than is the case with the universe of episodes of the body. We seem to have greater access to our bodies than to our minds via our intentions.

My conclusion here can be countered by the following argument. One must not be misled, the argument goes, by the superficial linguistic fact that words like 'understanding', 'loving', and 'desiring' behave like state-verbs from a grammatical point of view. Understanding, according to this argument, is a complicated process that involves an active decoding of messages or decoding of other external events as well as a restructuring of the decoded material into a form comprehensible to oneself. Likewise, love, hatred, and desire are not static states in the way a physical object's standing on the ground constitutes such a state. When one loves a person one can very well go through a very complicated and bewildering process, a process which may also entail a sequence of actions, such as approaching the object of one's love.

A lot of insight lies behind these points. However, we can still see a clear distinction between these mental episodes and the paradigm cases of intentional action. One cannot intend to understand, desire, and love and then just proceed to do so in the way one intends to go out for a walk and then just proceeds to act accordingly.

Back to my initial question. Do no intentional mental actions exist at all? Is the universe of the mind totally exhausted by states and uncontrolled streams of happenings? No, this is not so. Mental actions exist. I will, in the following, consider some prominent mental actions. I will proceed by viewing the mental faculties separately.

3.3.3 Cognitive abilities and cognitive actions

The most prominent of cognitive actions is thinking. At least many subspecies of thinking are intentional actions. One can intend to start thinking about one's finances or about a philosophical problem and then proceed to do so. Thinking is a very general category of action. Thinking has many important subspecies such as calculating, considering, reasoning, paying attention to, imagining.

Thinking is not only general in the sense that it has many subspecies. It is also general in the sense that it can take as objects all elements of the conceivable universe, concrete or abstract, and also all conceivable combinations of these elements. One can think about the universe as a whole, but one can also think about molecules and amoebas as well as all combinations of molecules and biological organisms that make up our known universe. Thus, thinking is by its nature the most multifaceted and creative of all human actions, be they mental or physical.

We have thus in the ability to think a paradigm case of mental ability in the sense of ability to perform an intentional mental action. This is of great relevance for our central topic. A person's capacity to think and also to think *correctly* or at least *rationally* (or reasonably correctly or rationally) is central to our idea of mental health. If this ability is severely reduced or otherwise disturbed we have a paradigm case of mental illness or mental disability.

Do other cognitive actions exist? Before answering this question I must again note that most of the cognitive concepts refer to states and not actions. I would like to offer the following preliminary list: knowing, being convinced, believing, understanding, seeing, hearing, feeling (perceptually), identifying, tasting, and smelling. All these states of affairs can happen to a person and typically occur without the subject intending to do anything in particular.

However, intentional mental actions exist that are *connected* to some of these states. An important category of such actions is of the type 'trying to F', 'putting oneself in the position to F', or 'seeing to it that one F's', where F is a mental state or process verb. Learning French means seeing to it that one knows French; listening to a speech means, at least partly, trying to hear it or seeing to it that one hears it.

3.3.4 **Emotive and conative abilities**

I will now consider the faculties of emotion and will. Here, the dominance of states over actions is even greater than in the case of the cognitive faculty. The emotions are per definition or in themselves *states* of emotion. Such is the case with love, hatred, envy, jealousy, happiness, contentment, distress, grief, and hope, just to mention a few types.

But could we not find parallels to the cognitive actions of 'trying to *F*' or 'setting oneself to *F*'? Can one not try to love Mrs Brown or try to hate Mr Smith? Can one not try to hope for the best or, indeed, can one not try to be happy? I think the answer differs here according to the type of emotion. Emotions are among themselves different in this respect. The key to this is the nature of the *object* of the emotion. By an object of an emotion I mean the object or the state of affairs to which the emotion is directed and which is a necessary condition for the occurrence of the emotion.

When I feel grateful I must believe that there is an object of my gratitude, namely a person who has done something good to me, for instance given me a present. This is a necessary condition for my gratitude. The necessity here is not only empirical, it is also conceptual. The concept of gratitude would not be properly used if it were not the case that the subject believed that someone else had done something good for him or her. Likewise, when I feel content-ment, some state of affairs must exist which I am content with, and which is according to my wants. If I did not want this state of affairs I could not, for conceptual reasons, be content with it.

Gratitude and contentment represent very different points on a continuum of emotions that is relevant here. The formal requirements of the object of gratitude are such that the subject cannot create them through an action of his or her own. Some other person must exist who has done a good thing for me to be grateful. Or, strictly speaking, I must *believe* that someone else has done the good thing for me. This is not the case with contentment, or with happi-ness, which is logically similar to contentment. People are typically content with things that they have achieved themselves. Therefore, hard work seems to be a good recipe for contentment. Here is also a good case for saying that one can through action create a state of emotion.

An important observation here is, though, that the action necessary for the realization of the emotional state is typically a physical action or a series of physical actions. Making oneself content does not have the character that learning, looking, or listening has in the cognitive case.

A few words can suffice concerning the will. The will is similar to emotions in the respect discussed here. To will is not to act, to want is not to act. One does not intend to will, nor does one intend to want something. One crucial and interesting exception exists, though, which deserves much more attention than I can direct to it here, and this is *the act of decision*. A decision is, as I have already argued, the act of creating an intention. And since intentions can be directed to all kinds of actions, decision has almost the same generality in the conative area as thinking has in the cognitive area.

A problem exists with regard to the act-character of decisions. I have argued that actions must per definition be intentional. Thus, when one decides one must intend to decide. But how does this intention come about? Is it also created through a decision? In such a case we end up in an infinite regress.

My answer is that no such regress is necessary. First, we can sustain the idea that decisions are intentional, but perhaps not very often consciously intentional. Clearly such cases exist though. A prime minister can express his intention to decide about a particular matter on the next day. And the next day he accordingly performs the act of decision. But although all decisions result in intentions, we have no reason to believe that all intentions come about as a result of decisions. This prevents the infinite regress.

3.3.5 A digression on an extended sense of mental abilities: abilities not related to actions. Consequences for the concept of health

The universe of mental *actions* is, at least concerning the most generic *types* of actions that there are, in a sense fairly poor. Thinking is the paradigm case of mental activity and some further cognitive actions exist which are more or less related to thinking. However, the emotive and conative areas, with the exception of decision, seem basically to lack action-types. What repercussion does this observation have upon a theory of mental health that is related to the notion of mental ability? Must mental health be reconstructed along lines different from those to be found in the case of somatic health?

As I noted at the beginning of this section, 'ability' need not be related to an intentional action: it may be synonymous with potentiality and refer to a disposition or liability. In this dispositional sense a person may, for instance, be able to grow or may be able to disintegrate, although neither of these processes is an intentional action.

Given this extension of the notion of ability, it seems as if all mental states and processes can be prefixed by ability. A man may be able to love a woman; a woman may be unable to hate or despise her fellow human beings; a child may be unable to feel remorse. The ability that we are talking about here is not the ability to perform a particular intentional mental action; it is rather the potentiality or the possibility of something's occurring. It is possible in the future that A will fall in love with a woman; it is, however, in our example, claimed to be impossible for the woman to start hating or despising someone or for the child to feel remorse.

One could then wonder whether my analysis of health has to be supplemented with a clause covering such mental abilities as are not directly related to intentional actions. It is evident, however, that defects with regard to such dispositions may enter into the characterization of psychiatric conditions. The subject who lacks the ability to be empathic or to fall in love lacks a disposition or a propensity. To cover such cases we might therefore propose the following generalization of the notion of health: A is completely healthy if, and only if, A has the second-order ability or the *general disposition* that is such that A can realize all his or her vital goals, given standard or accepted circumstances. The idea would then be, to take an example, that a person's health is reduced if he or she cannot fall in love with any other person, meaning that he or she has no propensity or disposition to fall in love.

Does a difficulty exist here? What if we generalize this idea to the physical universe? Suppose I replace 'ability to realize vital goals' with 'having the physical capacity to realize vital goals'? For instance, Sara is completely healthy only if she has the capacity to grow to a height that constitutes a vital goal for her. Or, John is completely healthy only if he has the capacity to retain his hair on his head throughout his life, if this constitutes a vital goal for him.

This is one way of proceeding but a completely different way of looking at the whole thing exists. This is to look at the non-intentional capacities as backgrounds for actions. A person who is not tall enough cannot become a basketball player, and maybe the playing of basketball is the more ultimate vital goal. Then, the basic natural capacity shows itself as a background for the relevant ability. One can conceive of a parallel analysis in the case of mental health. A person's incapacity for love or empathy may show itself in his or her inability to create lasting relationships with fellow human beings, which then is possibly a more ultimate vital goal for this person. Following this analysis we need not include the non-intentional capacities in the characterization of a person's health. They are, however, important when we characterize the *grounds* for the person's health.

A trouble then arises for the distinction between mental and somatic health. The creation of a lasting relationship cannot be characterized as a mental action. It is at least not a mental action in the strict sense with which I started my discussion: a mental action does not logically entail any particular physical event or state, apart from the existence of the agent. The distinction between mental and somatic health must then be found among the presuppositions or grounds for a person's ability to reach his or her vital goals. Probably this is the line to be followed in a further characterization of the distinction between the two kinds of health.

This conclusion can be reinforced when we study a wider spectrum of mental disorders than the ones that directly involve reduced mental abilities such as incoherent thinking or mental possibilities such as being able to fall in love. Consider instead the states of depression and anxiety. Both are mental states. But they do not just concern and affect mental actions or mental abilities. Depression and anxiety are mental states that block the performance of most kinds of actions, mental as well as physical. But if melancholic disorders and anxiety disorders (which are the terms in the formal *DSM* terminology) are to be classified as mental disorders, then the criterion cannot be the fact that they peculiarly involve reduced mental abilities. The criterion must be that the disabilities typical for these disorders have peculiarly mental causes, namely the mental states of depression and anxiety.

3.3.6 **On mental abilities and their opportunities**

Before concluding I will add a word of caution. The notions of possibility and impossibility (as unqualified) entail all kinds of conditions for something occurring or not occurring. These kinds of conditions can be both of an internal and an external kind. In the general theory of action, presented above, this distinction is often indicated by using the terms 'ability' and 'opportunity'. A person needs both ability and an opportunity for a particular action to be performed. The person may be able to learn French but will perhaps never learn French because there is never an opportunity. No course in French may be available in the town where this person lives, or he or she will never have the time to learn French.

In the case of physical action the opportunities very often have to do with external circumstances. With mental actions or mental states the scenario is slightly different. In a way mental episodes seem independent of the external world. One seems to be able to think independently of any configuration of facts outside oneself. We are mistaken, however, if we believe that mental episodes completely lack such dependence. All actions and all episodes that need some concentration or effort on the part of the agent can be disturbed and in the extreme case be extinguished by external circumstances. For instance, one cannot think properly if someone or something seriously disturbs one's concentration. Clearly, many emotions and moods also require peaceful and quiet surroundings.

We can conclude, then, that most (perhaps all) mental episodes require some opportunity for their existence. This means that the standard distinction between ability and opportunity in action theory can and should be brought over to the theory of mental episodes, not only the theory of mental actions.

I have argued elsewhere that ability, in contradistinction to opportunity, is the core notion in the general theory of health. Health has to do with a person's inner resources, not with external circumstances. I wish to argue in a similar way about mental health. We do not consider a person mentally unhealthy on the ground that he or she is unable to think correctly because of being continuously disturbed. The person may be mentally unhealthy, though, on the ground that he or she cannot think under standard or reasonable circumstances.

3.3.7 Concluding words

My task in this section has been to scrutinize the notion of mental action and mental ability with, in the end, the notion of mental health in mind. As a guide for analysis, I have then used my own general notion of health that is formulated in terms of a person's ability to realize vital goals. I have noted that the universe of mental intentional actions is not very large. It seems therefore implausible to base the notions of mental health and mental disorder on the idea of a person's ability (or inability) to perform intentional mental actions. The primary category to be targeted by such a notion would be abilities or inabilities to think or to think coherently. But this category covers only a limited part of mental health and mental disorder.

In a second step I have tried to extend my characterization of health to deal not only with abilities to perform intentional actions but also with general propensities and possibilities with regard to entering certain states. Although such a notion would have a wider scope, including people's propensities or possibilities with regard to having a rich emotional life, it would still fall short of an all-inclusive characterization of mental health. I used the conditions of depression and anxiety as examples of mental disorders that are not covered by such a notion.

A much more plausible candidate for the characterization of mental disorder in general would therefore be that the disabilities typical for these disorders have peculiarly *mental causes*, for instance, the mental states of depression and anxiety.

In the study of mental disorder, later in this book, I will not attempt to give a general characterization. Instead I will focus on a crucial subcategory where irrationality and compulsion are the central notions. (For an interesting analysis of mental disorders as disorders that can be understood in terms of reasons, see Matthews 2003.)

Chapter 4

On the understanding and explanation of actions

4.1 Introduction

So far I have attempted to characterize the notion of action from various angles. I will now briefly turn to the clarification of explanation of actions. A full version of this presentation exists in my *Action, Ability and Health* (2000).

An explanation can be an answer to several questions, the most salient being what-, how- and why-questions. One can explain what something is by describing its inner nature and its functions. One can explain how something functions by following the details in the process that constitutes the functioning. Finally, one explains why an event occurs by connecting this event with some other event(s), mainly among such events as precede the one to be explained.

In the case of actions, the what- and the why-questions are highly relevant. I will distinguish between the answers given to these questions by using the terms 'understanding' for the what-questions and 'explanation' for the why-questions. This is an idiosyncratic use of these terms. Many prominent philosophers of action use them in other ways. (See, for instance, Ricoeur 1981.)

The main bulk of my analysis will be focused on explanation of action. The explanation, however, presupposes some understanding. I will therefore first present my view of the understanding of action.

4.2 On understanding actions

What does it mean to give an answer to the question 'what is this'? in relation to actions? Assume that two persons (*A* and *B*) witness the occurrence of a behaviour performed by a man *C*. Assume that they witness *C* is waving his hand. *A* asks *B* what is going on.

B's first task is to identify the performance as an action in the first place. The context is not legal, so *B* can wholly concentrate on the issue of intentionality. Does this behaviour issue from some intention of *C*'s? *B*'s task is one of interpretation. The answer is not self-evident since the intention in question, being a mental event, is not observable. *B* has to find evidence for assuming the existence of the intention. Different methods for this exist. If *C* is approachable for questioning one can simply ask him what he is doing. This is a recommendable procedure in many instances. However, it is not waterproof. C may lie about his intentions. He may deny any intentionality, and he may be mistaken about his true intentions. (See von Wright 1971.) A second task is therefore to put C's behaviour in a context. Where does the waving take place? Is there a human being in the neighbourhood to whom the waving can be directed? Is there anybody else doing the same thing as C?

Further observation by B may detect the following circumstances. C is standing together with a number of other people, all waving their hands, in front of a building. In a window on the upper floor of the building a man is standing looking at all the people outside. It is evident that the group outside are calling this person's attention to something. Thus, the primary question can be answered: C's behaviour is intentional. It is an action.

Preliminarily, B can now identify C's action as an action of waving. So far we do not know whether this identification is the adequate one. The people surrounding C have presumably a further purpose, i.e. they are not simply waving their hands. They intend to do something more. Possibly, though, there is a secondary (transmitted) intention to be described as the intention to wave the hand.

In the absence of reliable answers from any of the people involved, B needs a further contextual scrutiny. B may observe the place where all this is going on. The people are standing outside a government building. In the window they are calling on somebody whom B recognizes as the prime minister of Sweden. B happens to know that the government has decided just a day before to considerably raise the taxes on housing. Many houseowners, in particular in the capital where houses are expensive, are as a result outraged. Thus, it had been expected that they would protest in some way. B can also see that some of the people in the crowd are carrying posters with exclamations referring to the taxation. Hence, the identification of C's action seems to be complete. C is protesting to the prime minister against the government's proposal regarding house taxation. B can provide an adequate answer to A regarding the question: what is C doing?

To understand an action (in my technical sense of understand) is thus to correctly identify the action. A correct identification (at least outside the legal context) entails getting hold of the intention with which the agent acted (cf. Chapter 1, Section 1.5). In our example, C intended to protest by waving a poster in front of the prime minister. Thus, the action performed by C is one of protesting.

A problem arising here is the following. As we have seen above, a person normally has more than one intention in an action situation (through intention transmission). Which intention is then the action-characterizing one?

It is tempting to say, and I have already preliminarily alluded to this, that the action-characterizing intention is the ultimate intention behind the action. If C intends to protest and nothing further, then the action is one of protest. If C intends to greet a person by waving his hand, then the action is one of greeting. (For similar conclusions, see Chapter 1, Section 1.5, on the description of actions.)

But we have already seen in the section on rationality and norms above that a further reason may exist behind an action. This reason can be used in *explaining* the action in question. I will illustrate by further analysing the protest case. One may ask, why does C protest to the prime minister? A natural answer is that C does not want to be ruined; he wishes to survive. This wish to survive has issued in a decision to fight for survival. But why, then, is the action not to be described as the action of fighting for survival? Let me illustrate with the example used when I introduced the notion of intention transmission. The man who travels to Tokyo certainly has some good reason for travelling to Tokyo. He may want to sign a contract with a company in Japan. This want has issued in a decision to sign a contract. But why, then, is his action not to be described as the action of signing a contract in Japan?

These questions are tricky. What they point to is that the intention to be chosen for identifying an action cannot be the ultimate intention in the chain of intention transmission. If this were so there would be no place for action-explanation in terms of further reasons and intentions. Moreover, there would be quite a few actions, if they were all to be described in terms of the ultimate intentions.

I doubt that we can find a single final answer to this question. Probably the answer must be pragmatic and related to a particular discourse. A good rule of thumb would be to find the level on which the agent him- or herself identifies the action performed. There may, however, be contexts where an observer may have good arguments for identifying the action in a slightly different way, either on a lower or on a higher level of abstraction.

However, for many purposes some level must be found: it is crucial to identify an action somewhere. This is particularly salient in the context of explanation, when we set out to answer the question *why* an action has been performed. An answer to the question 'why?' presupposes an identification of that which is to be explained. This brings me to the issue of action-explanation.

4.3 On explanation of actions

4.3.1 Introduction

In what ways are actions normally explained? What do we normally refer to when we try to explain why a particular action has been performed? If one looks at ordinary language, one will find a varied collection of locutions used for the purpose of explaining actions. The following list may perhaps contain the most important types:

I. Explanations of actions by reference to a mental property of the agent:

    (i) by reference to the agent's *intentions* or *aims* ('*A* went into the bookshop because she intended to buy a book' or simply 'went into the bookshop in order to buy a book');

    (ii) by reference to the agent's *beliefs* ('*A* closed the window because she believed that it was going to rain');

    (iii) by reference to the agent's *wants* ('*A* killed her neighbour because she wanted to marry the neighbour's husband');

    (iv) by reference to the agent's *emotions* ('*A* hit her son because she was angry with him');

    (v) by reference to the agent's *attitudes or character traits* ('*A* worked hard because she was ambitious');

    (vi) by reference to the agent's *sensations* ('*A* walked up and down because she was in great pain');

    (vii) by reference to the agent's *perceptions* ('*A* called for the ambulance because she had observed a car-crash').

II. Explanations of actions by reference to a fact external to the agent:

    (viii) by reference to an *external episode* ('*A* jumped on to the pavement because there was a car coming towards her');

    (ix) by reference to *compulsion* ('*A* handed over the bank's money because a robber forced her to');

    (x) by reference to a *norm* ('*A* thanked the hostess for the dinner, because that is the norm in Swedish society').

This is just a provisional and superficial classification indicated by ordinary locutions. An examination of the listed examples will enable me to make another and more enlightening systematization. Let me just insert a note concerning the terms 'motive' and 'reason'. These are terms very often used in action-explanations. In the following, I shall completely avoid the term 'motive'. The main reason for this is that ordinary language seems to permit us to refer to practically any explanatory factor of an action as its motive. Intentions, wants, emotions, and attitudes can all in most contexts be referred to as motives when they occur in explanatory contexts. Sometimes external facts are also called motives.

The same observation applies to a great extent to 'reason'. There is, however, a fairly clear, more narrow use of 'reason', where reasons are contrasted with intentions and wants and taken to refer (primarily) to facts external to the agents. In this section, I shall adopt this more narrow concept of reason and use the term 'rational explanation' for explanation in terms of such facts. (In Part 2, however, I will use a broader notion of reason, including wants.)

4.3.2 A schema for intentional explanation

I have elsewhere argued at length (2000) that all the mentioned kinds of action-explanation have a common ultimate analysis. The core notion in this analysis is the concept of *intention*. It can be shown that all the mentioned explanation types are elliptic variants of – as I shall call it – a complete intentional explanation, using a *complete intentional explanans*.

The structure of this explanation is the following:

(i) *A* intends to bring about *P*

(ii) *A* believes that he or she is in situation *C*

(iii) *A* believes that *A* will not bring about *P* in *C* unless *A* does *F*

(iv) *A* can do *F* in *C*

(v) *A* sets him- or herself to do *F*

(i)–(iv) constitute together what I will call a *complete intentional explanans* of (v). (This schema will also be referred to as a practical syllogism *PSI*, see below.) What I mean by this is that the fact that *A* sets him- or herself to do *F* is in a way completely explained by referring to *A*'s intention, *A*'s two kinds of beliefs and *A*'s practical possibility. This contention concerning completeness must not be misunderstood. It does not rule out other, more distant explanations of the same action, in terms of, for instance, the agent's ideology or some environmental influence. What is considered complete here is only the most proximate *explanans*. The intentional *explanans* contains those factors that in time are the most proximate *explanantia* of the action to be explained.

Before applying this model of action-explanation to the analysis of a variety of explanations in ordinary language and human sciences, I will attempt to answer a criticism which is sometimes raised against it. This criticism concerns the scope of the model: it claims that the model has too strong presuppositions concerning the nature of human action to have any practical implications; in particular, it claims that the model presupposes that the agent whose action is to be explained is an ideally rational person.

This criticism misunderstands what the analysis of the intentional *explanans* entails. The *explanans* does *not* present the thinking of an ideally rational agent. Observe that nothing is presupposed about the rationality or the quality of the beliefs contained in the second and third premises of the *explanans*. The beliefs may be false and they may be the consequence of incoherent thinking.

Similarly, the intention contained in the *explanans* may be counter-productive with regard to the agent's ultimate purposes. The agent may, for instance, through incoherent reasoning have come to the conclusion that a particular state of affairs is an appropriate means for realizing the ultimate purpose despite its not actually being so.

Thus the *explanans* does not express any rationality on the part of the agent. What the *explanans* entails is the following: Given that premises of types 1–4 are true, then for logical reasons a conclusion of type 5 must be true. In other words, given that an agent has an intention and a certain set of beliefs, and given that the agent is capable and unprevented, then he or she must act in a certain direction. If the agent does not act, then something must be wrong with one or more of the premises. Either it cannot be true that the agent *really* intends, or it cannot be true that the agent *really* believes what he or she is claimed to believe, or, finally, that the agent is not capable or unprevented. (In Nordenfelt 2000, I have presented further arguments for this logical deduction thesis.)

By way of summary: my model for the intentional *explanans* is not exclusively an analysis of the explanation of rational action: it is an analysis of the conceptual structure of intending, believing, and being able to act. (See von Wright 1976, pp. 409–410, for a discussion of this issue.)

4.3.3 The relation between intentional and causal explanations

It is well known that intentional or rational explanations were the subject of much controversy in the 1960s and 1970s in the English-speaking philosophical world. There was discussion about whether an intentional or rational explanation constituted a causal explanation or some kind of logical explanation of the action in question.

A starting point for this discussion was the analysis proposed by the logical positivists, in particular Carl Hempel (1965). Hempel argued that a scientific explanation (including causal explanations) must consist of the following elements: a universal law premise, an initial condition premise, and the *explanandum*. The latter follows logically from the two premises. Formally:

$$L1 \dots Ln$$
$$\underline{C1 \dots Cn}$$
$$E$$

The *explanandum* should be deducible from the two premises. The model thus described is the famous deductive-nomological model of explanation. This model has been followed by several slightly different versions, some of which contain probabilistic laws instead of universal deterministic laws. A common feature of the various *explanantia*, however, is that they contain some law-like premises.

A number of writers with a humanistic inclination contested the applicability of this model, in any of its versions, to the explanation of human actions. They said that there is something special about explanations of human actions because there is a peculiar relation between the typical *explanantia* of human actions and the actions themselves. A typical *explanans* of a human action, they said, is an intention or a reason. One explains why a person does something by referring to his or her intentions or reasons. This kind of explanation, the argument goes, is not an ordinary causal explanation of the kind that we meet in the sciences. An intention or a reason cannot be a cause of the action that it explains.

The latter crucial contention is in its turn backed up by different arguments from different authors. The historian Dray (1957) focused on reasons and what he called rational explanations. He claimed that the most significant feature of a rational action-explanation is that it shows the *appropriateness* of the action to be explained. This distinguishes rational explanations from causal explanations. When one explains the movement of a billiard ball by citing its cause, one does not in any sense show the appropriateness of the movement of the ball. (For a response, see Hempel 1963.) Other authors, for example Melden (1961) and von Wright (1971), have advanced the thesis that the relation between the intention and the intended action is in some sense logical. And a logical connection between the two entities, they say, excludes an empirical causal connection between the two entities.

Moreover, the humanistic theorists claim, there is in an explanation of action hardly ever any reference, explicit or implicit, to a universal law. When one explains why Peter does something, one does not normally refer to any information about how people who are similar to Peter behave in a similar situation. Instead one wants to know further things about Peter, what he intended in the situation in question, what he knew or believed about possible means to fulfil his intention. In short, according to the humanistic lines of reasoning, intentional or rational explanations are non-causal and non-Hempelian. These explanations are peculiar and distinct from ordinary scientific explanations.

I will in the following attempt to show how my analysis of the notion of an intention can provide a bridge between these two camps in the theory of explanation. The notion of a *disposition* is a key factor in my argument. My whole analysis relies on the hypothesis that intentions can be viewed as a species of dispositions. Consider first a simple kind of disposition, namely brittleness, and an explanation in terms of it. We wish, for instance, to explain that a window breaks by referring to its dispositional property brittleness and, in addition, to the fact that something hard hit the window.

An explanation of the fact that the window breaks can then be put in the following way: The window breaks because it was hit by a hard object *and* because of that property of the window, viz. brittleness, which is such that if the window is hit by a hard object, then it breaks. In this formulation it is evident that the *explanandum* follows logically from the *explanans*. The logical structure is the following:

$$Fa \rightarrow Ga$$
$$\underline{Fa}$$
$$Ga$$

We observe that this is an explanation that is deductive in form, hence fulfilling one of Hempel's requirements regarding an explanation. However, it is not deductive in virtue of the existence of a universal law. It is deductive in virtue of a dispositional hypothetical.

This, then, is in principle the simple logic that can be applied to the intentional explanatory schema put forward above. I have in fact proposed a dispositional analysis of intentions, and it is easy to show that the schema of intentional explanation is deductive in the way an explanation according to the ordinary dispositional paradigm is. With regard to details the situation is slightly more complicated when it comes to intentions. In the simple dispositional paradigm, the consequent of the hypothetical is identical with the conclusion of the argument. In the intentional case there is normally no direct reference to the action to be explained. One intends to attain a goal, a state of affairs P, and finally one performs an action F distinct from P but which is believed to be conducive to P.

An intention, as my analysis has suggested, is a disposition not just to perform a single action but to perform a number of actions, namely all those actions which the agent believes to be necessary for the achievement of the intended state. Hence in the intentional analysis we need some universal quantification, which is absent from the simple dispositional paradigm. But observe: this does not transform the expression into a universal law. The expression still refers to a particular agent A and no other agent; it is only that A is disposed to perform more than one action when A has an intention. A is disposed to perform *all* actions which have a particular property.

From this reasoning the following conclusions can be drawn:

(i) The schema of intentional explanation has the form of a deductive logical argument.

(ii) It contains no universal law, however. It is deductive in virtue of the existence of a dispositional hypothetical.

(iii) But since dispositional explanations occur outside the field of action-explanations, the intentional explanatory schema is in a sense reduced to a kind of explanation that is not peculiar to the humanities.

It could now, however, be asked what implication this solution has for the anti-causal idea. Does it still mean that intentions are not causes as the proponents of the logical connection argument insist? The question requires a careful answer. I shall now first give only a partial answer, then return to the issue in replying to an objection to my theory. It should here be borne in mind that in the intentional explanation, as reconstructed by me, I do not use the whole content of what it means to have an intention. As I have mentioned earlier, to intend also means to believe that one can realize the intended end. This information is not necessary for the deduction of our *explanandum*. There may be other elements contained in the analysis of '*A* intends to bring about *P*'. Likewise, there are other elements than the ones used in a dispositional explanation contained in the full analysis of, for instance, 'this window is brittle'.

This should be borne in mind because the answer that I give now concerns only that part of the analysis of dispositions and intentions that is contained in the explanatory arguments, namely the hypotheticals. And the question can now be framed: Can a hypothetical fact be a cause?

How do we look upon things in the case of a Hempelian explanatory argument (e.g. Hempel 1965)? What things are causes and what are not causes among the premises in this argument? If we deal with a Hempelian reconstruction of a causal explanation it is obvious that the cause or causes are the factors that are put among the initial conditions. The universal law itself, the universal hypothetical, is not a cause, although it is of course one of the premises in the Hempelian reconstruction of a causal explanation. Likewise in a dispositional explanation, in general, it is the second premise, or that which is signified by the second premise, which is considered to be the cause. In our brittleness case, it is the fact that the window is hit that is the cause. The hypothetical fact used in the dispositional explanation is not of the right category to be a cause. Hence the answer to our question whether the dispositional hypothetical is a cause is: no. This means also that the *intentional* hypothetical is not of the right type to be a cause.

This conclusion, however, does not have anything to do with a logical-connection argument. It is a conclusion based on considerations about the ontological status of laws and hypothetical facts. (One ought to be able to distinguish between that which is a cause and that which the cause is a cause in virtue of, namely a law or a dispositional hypothetical. In (2000) I in fact coined the term 'semi-universal law' for this dispositional hypothetical fact.) But observe, again, that the hypothetical is not the whole analysis of the disposition. The hypothetical is true in virtue of a categorical fact. Nothing prevents this categorical fact from being a cause and from playing the role of an initial condition in a deductive nomological or dispositional explanation of the same *explanandum*. (Compare this analysis with my presentation of Bolton's analysis of the mind-body relation in Chapter 1, Section 1.4.)

4.4 The relation between wants and intentions: a practical syllogism of wants

If one replaces 'intend' by 'want' in the schema one gets something that under no circumstances is a valid argument. First, *A*'s want to do *F* is compatible with *A*'s believing that he cannot do *F*. Second, *A*'s want to do *F* is compatible with his having a conflicting want to do *non-F*. (The concept of intention, in my present interpretation, excludes the existence of subjectively conflicting intentions.) Thus, *A*'s doing *F* need not at all follow from his want to do *F*, even if *A* is capable and unprevented. There is still, however, I shall contend, a strong connection between wants and intentions. I wish to propose that a want is also a kind of disposition. *A person who has a want to do F has ipso facto a disposition to form an intention to do F.* This disposition has among its antecedents the kind of factors just mentioned. Thus, a person who wants to go out for a walk has a disposition to form the intention to go out for a walk, which will be realized, given that he has no overriding conflicting want and that he believes that he can go out for a walk. Sometimes, the forming of an intention is an action on the part of the agent. This action is called a *decision*. Intentions can, however, come about, I will assume, without being preceded by a decision.

In the subsequent chapter on deliberation of action I will make substantial use of a practical syllogism including wants instead of intentions.

4.5 The intentional explanatory schema applied

It can now be shown, and this is of importance both for the theory of explanation and for the theory of determination of action, that the explanatory schema can incorporate and explicate most instances of *all* the following action-explanations occurring in ordinary speech and in science: explanations in terms of intentions, beliefs, abilities, opportunities, wants, emotions, attitudes and character traits, sensations, perceptions, external reasons, and compulsion.

I have elsewhere (2000) demonstrated this thesis with all the mentioned categories. I will here confine myself to giving the basic arguments for my general contention and illustrate with a few of the categories.

4.5.1 Explanations in terms of intentions, beliefs, abilities, and opportunities

It is easy to see that ordinary explanations in terms of intentions, beliefs, abilities, and opportunities are only incomplete variants of the complete intentional *explanans*. Consider the following examples: (i) *A* went into the bookshop because she intended to buy a certain book. (ii) *A* went into the bookshop because she believed that the book was to be found there. (iii) *A* went into the bookshop because she believed that she had to do that in order to find the book. (iv) *A* went into the bookshop because she was capable of and unprevented from doing so.

Together these colloquial explanations form a complete intentional *explanans*. In a situation when only one is quoted it is easily seen that the others must be presupposed. When (i) is explicitly given (ii)–(iv) are implicitly taken to be the case. When (ii) is explicitly given (i), (iii), and (iv) are implicitly taken to be the case, etc. When, for instance we say that A went into the bookshop because she believed that a book was to be found there, we must certainly presuppose that she intended to get hold of this book and that she thought it was necessary to actually enter the shop in order to get hold of it.

4.5.2 Explanations in terms of perceptions and reasons: rational explanation

Actions are frequently explained, not by reference to any mental property of the agent but by reference to a fact external to the agent. Consider the following example: 'A jumped on to the pavement because a car was coming towards her'. How is the relation between such an external fact and the human action to be analysed?

An external event cannot be treated in the way that I have proposed for intentions and wants. No conditional element is present in it; it cannot be treated as a disposition. The temptation is then great to assume that the relation between an external fact and an action in the case where the former explains the latter is in a straightforward way causal.

Many contemporary philosophers have, however, firmly denied that this can be the case. A *reason* they claim, does not explain in the way that a cause does. In an analysis of an explanation in terms of reasons (or a rational explanation), we must take account of the peculiar relation that holds between the notions of reason and intention. No analogous relation, they say, exists between cause and intention.

In the treatment that I propose, I will attempt to explicate the nature of the relation between reasons, intentions, and actions. A reason is an explanatory factor that is, in contradistinction to most causes, a part of an intentional *explanans* or, in certain cases, a want *explanans*. More specifically, the reason, or strictly speaking the agent's awareness of the reason, constitutes the fulfilment of the second element of the intentional explanatory schema, the *PSI*.

I will first analyse the concrete case. How could it be that the car's coming towards *A* 'made' *A* jump on to the pavement? One trivial but necessary condition was that *A* became aware of the fact (or at least believed it to be a fact) that the car was approaching her. Another necessary condition was that *A* judged the situation to be what it was and judged the consequences it was likely to have – in short that *A* believed the situation to be dangerous. If *A* did not believe that the car was dangerous and that it would probably kill her, the observation of the car would obviously have nothing to do with the explanation of *A*'s movements.

This is not enough. No action would be performed by *A* in this situation unless *A* intended to achieve something. *A* would not have moved unless *A* had had the intention (at least) to survive. If *A* had been in a mood where *A* did not care about her life or health, the observation of the dangerous car would not have incited *A* to react in the way she did. (I am of course here presupposing that we are not dealing with a pure reflex movement.) Since *A*, however, intended to preserve the state of being alive, *A* consequently set herself to jump out of the way. To jump away was, as *A* correctly judged, a necessary and sufficient condition for staying alive, given the circumstances surrounding her. Consider the case schematically:

(i) A car is coming towards *A* (the reason).

(ii) *A* becomes aware of (i) and judges it to be what it is.

(iii) *A* intends to avoid being killed.

(iv) *A* believes that she is going to get killed in the circumstances surrounding her, unless *A* jumps on to the pavement.

(v) *A* is capable of and not prevented from jumping on to the pavement.

(vi) *A* jumps on to the pavement.

Given this analysis we can see that the components nicely fit the pattern of the intentional explanation. *The reason is identical with that circumstance which, when perceived by the agent, is considered by him or her to make a certain course of action necessary in order to achieve or preserve an intended end.* The reason, then, is to be found in the second component of the intentional *explanans*. The fact that the agent perceives or otherwise becomes aware of the reason constitutes the whole second component of the *explanans*.

According to this analysis, a rational explanation is another elliptic way of explaining an action. It is now easily seen that the explanation 'Jane jumped on to the pavement because she *saw* a car approaching her', i.e. an explanation in terms of a perception, follows exactly the same pattern.

4.5.3 Summary

We have found that explanations of actions in terms of intentions, beliefs, abilities, opportunities, and external reasons may all be incomplete variants of intentional explanation. They are, however, variants incomplete in slightly different ways: in the case of the first four categories they entail the explicit mentioning of one of the four factors in a complete intentional *explanans*; in the case of external reasons the explicit factor is a part of the second factor in the *explanans*, namely the circumstance that the agent believes to be the case.

4.6 A critique of the classical model: John Searle

In an extremely interesting book, *Rationality in Action* (2001), John Searle has written a vigorous critique of what he calls the classical model of rationality and of the relations between, on the one hand, desires, intentions, and reasons and, on the other hand, the actions desired, intended, and reasoned. Since I find myself to be a proponent of a version of the classical model I feel provoked to reply to Searle's critique. (Since I have read Searle's book at quite a late stage in the production of my own text my comments take the form of an appendix to my main analysis.)

According to a simple classical model, says Searle, desires, intentions, and reasons can be sufficient causes of actions. They can cause actions in the same way as billiard balls can cause other billiard balls to move and they can be sufficient causes in the same way as billiard balls can. This, however, Searle argues, is an unreasonable way of looking at the connection between actions and their antecedents. Intentions, desires, and reasons do not cause in this mechanical way. Instead it is the person's *self* that chooses to let them operate. Searle says: 'The question why did you do that? does not ask: what causes were sufficient to determine your actions? But rather it asks: what reasons did you as a rational self, act on'? (pp. 85–86).

Searle introduces the notion of a *gap*. He says that there are gaps in a person's decision procedures. There is a gap between a desire and an intention, between an intention and the starting of an action and also between an intention and the continuation of an action. At every stage we need something over and above the mentioned antecedent to bring about the consequent. This something, according to Searle, is the person's own choice. The person lets the desire result in an intention and the person chooses to act on the ground of an intention. So, at every stage there is a self who acts on the ground of desires,

intentions, and reasons. The mental antecedents are not in themselves sufficient causes.

Searle thus advances three theses:

1. We have experiences of the gap of the sort I have described.
2. We have to presuppose the gap. We have to presuppose that the psycholog-
    ical antecedents of many of our decisions and actions do not set causally
    sufficient conditions for those decisions and actions.
3. In normal conscious life one cannot avoid choosing and deciding.

I think Searle's reasoning is quite strong and that it deserves careful attention,
but I will not here engage in an argument with him. Instead, I will confine
myself to finding out to what extent I have been endorsing the classical model
and, in particular, whether this endorsement together with Searle's critique
undermines my main observations and my classification of action-explanations.

First, I am not an exponent of the simplest form of a classical model. I have
analysed wants and intentions in terms of dispositions to actions and not as
causes *tout court*. On the other hand, this does not help me much. The conditional that serves as *analysans* of the disposition is an ordinary causal conditional. For instance, given that a subject has an intention then, according to
my analysis, this subject is in a state such that if he or she believes that something is the case then he or she will act. There is no gap indicated here. There is
no place for further choice. Thus my theory is a classical theory.

On the other hand, I have in an early exposition of my theory of action-
explanation (1974, pp. 84–85) implicitly acknowledged the existence of the
self and let it play a crucial role in the determination of action. (I did not then,
however, pay further attention to this fact.) There I discussed the fact that an
intentional disposition may seem peculiar in the sense that it may not be
released until late after its formation. When I say that I intend to travel to Paris
next June I have formed an intention that will not immediately result in
action. The action will not be performed, under normal circumstances, before
June. I note, however, that this is nothing peculiar to intentions. There are
many other dispositions that have delayed action. Consider, for instance, a
primed bomb. Assume that we have primed a bomb to go off in 48 hours.
Then this bomb has a disposition that is such that it will not act upon it until
48 hours later. Something can happen with the bomb before the action. In
particular, the bomb can be deprimed at some stage before it goes off. Then
the bomb loses its disposition. Likewise, I argue, I can *drop my intention* to go
to Paris. I can change my mind. This means that the causal conditional constituted by my intention is only a provisional one. It is a causal conditional as
long as I let it be there. Thus, I admit a stratification of the mind such that

there is always a self who ultimately monitors the performance of the actions in question.

Thus, when I intend to do something then I have only for the time being committed myself to this doing. I will perform the action in question provided I discover no reason to change my mind. My expressions are slightly different than Searle's and he would probably say that the self does not just let an intention be released. The self instead *acts on* the intention.

However that may be, I have in fact, like Searle, admitted that the intention (or the desire or the reason) is not a sufficient but only a partial cause of the action intended (desired or reasoned). Does this acknowledgement have crucial repercussions on my previous (and coming) analysis of action determination? I do not think so. As long as we admit that the causal conditionals constituting the mental antecedents of action are provisional and can be removed, the analysis of the concepts can, I think, remain substantially unchanged. An intention can still for many purposes be viewed as a causal conditional which, given the assent of the agent, will result in an action. (For a sophisticated recent analysis of decision-making relevant to this discussion, see Stroud 2003.)

Part 2

Irrationality, Compulsion, and Mental Disorder

Chapter 5

Reasons for action and rationality

5.1 **Introduction**

This second part of the essay will be focused more on issues of direct relevance to psychiatry. I will deal at length with issues of rationality and differentiate between various kinds of rationality and irrationality. In order to make these distinctions, I will make substantial use of the action-theoretic background presented in Part 1, in particular the analysis of intentional and rational explanation. At a later stage, I will focus on the notion of compulsion, which I take to be particularly central to the systematic study of particular psychiatric disorders. I will attempt to show that compulsion is also a variant of intentional determination. Finally, I will use the notions of rationality and compulsion to study some examples of mental disorders.

My more specific purpose in this part of the book is the following. I will first analyse what could be considered to be a perfect or ideal rationalization of an action. What conditions should be fulfilled in a perfect deliberation? From there, I have the possibility of discerning all the ways in which a deliberation can go wrong from the point of view of this ideal. Many possibilities for such defects exist. All human beings fall short of the ideal in some respect. Very few of these shortcomings, however, need indicate the presence of any pathology.

Here, the criteria of health come in. The reason why many forms of irrationality do not matter is that they do not prevent us from dealing with our daily affairs in an acceptable way. Only when the irrationality really becomes a hindrance, when it disrupts daily life, do we have a point in saying that it constitutes an illness.

Mental illnesses or disorders (I will mostly use the term 'disorder', thereby complying with the praxis in the *Diagnostic and Statistical Manual of Mental Disorders [DSM-IV]*) are, to a great extent, connected with deviant behaviour and with inability to act properly. Although this is a salient fact, it has so far prompted little systematic investigation into the mechanisms of such deviancy and disability. (Pears 1984, and Charlton 1988, are two who have conducted such investigation.) The disability involved in mental disorder does not normally have a clear somatic background, as in the case of a broken leg or the exhausted body that is ravaged by serious infection or cancer. The basis of mental disorder has rather to do with the volitional and emotional machinery of action, with the person's intentions and reasons and with his or her moods and emotions, which in turn determine the person's intentions and reasons.

Philosophical action theory now has a conceptual apparatus that is rich enough to allow for the formulation of hypotheses concerning the defective machinery of mental illness. One author – a philosopher and psychiatrist – has started exploring this area in a very efficient way. This author is Fulford, who, particularly in his *Moral Theory and Medical Practice* (1989), has proposed a general theory of mental health in action-theoretic terms. He has also, particularly in the area of delusions, suggested a more detailed analysis of notions such as reason and intention for the purpose of characterizing various mental illnesses.

In his book, Fulford introduced the idea that delusions should be viewed not, as in traditional accounts, as false beliefs or unjustified beliefs, but instead as *defective reasons for action*. In putting forward this suggestion, he has behind him some moral support from prominent psychiatrists, for instance Mullen (1979), who in his *Phenomenology of Disordered Mental Function* says (p. 40): 'Delusion represents a profound and complex disorganization of mental life, stretching way beyond mere false ideas and mistaken beliefs'. One of the reasons behind Fulford's more specific idea is that a delusion need not be of the belief-kind at all; it could instead be a value-judgment, for instance the expression of an extremely odd desire. (It appears that Fulford includes expressions of desires and needs among value-judgments.) Reasons for action can be both of the belief-kind and of the desire-kind. Fulford, therefore, finds it plausible to assume that the distinctive feature of a delusion is that the delusion is not a false or unjustified belief but some other defect in a human being's practical reasoning, for instance a defective reason for action. His idea, then, is that neither the desires nor the beliefs or the factual judgments should, as such, be counted as delusions. Instead, it is in their *capacities* as reasons for action that we find the distinctively delusive character of the desires, beliefs, and factual judgments. I quote:

> Neither all factual judgments nor all value judgments are reasons for action. Hence, something different from or over and above their status, respectively, as factual judgments or as value judgments, is required to mark out either *as* a reason for action. Hence, if delusions are or are derived from defective reasons for action, it is in this 'something different from or over and above' that their defectiveness would be located. (Fulford 1989, p. 216)

I find this idea intriguing, and this has led me to initiate an investigation into the notion of a defective reason for action. My general conclusion entails a rather special interpretation of Fulford's suggestions. Delusions certainly function as reasons for action. They normally rationalize actions perfectly well in the light of the machinery I will spell out. They could, however, be said to be defective in the sense that they are often alien elements in the mind of the subject. They often stand out in relation to other beliefs or evaluations that the subject has. Moreover, they normally function as *compelling* reasons for the actions they rationalize.

In order to substantiate this conclusion, I make a long digression into the notion of compulsion, trying to demonstrate the following: the factor that is really disturbing to the subject in mental disorders such as schizophrenia, paranoia, and obsession, and what makes them prevent the subject from realizing his or her vital goals, is not so much that they tend to lead to irrational actions. The crucial factor is that the subject is *unable to avoid* performing the irrational action. The subject is or feels compelled to act in the way he or she does.

Accordingly, it will become obvious that some of the interpretations of the notion of defective rationality that I will present have little or no relation to psychiatry. Then, the investigation may, however, serve the purpose of identifying the relevance of the notion of defective reason to the theory of delusions. My analysis in this part can also be looked upon as a treatise in its own right, quite independently of its relation to psychiatry. The theory of action in itself provides sufficient reason for studying systematically the ways in which reasons for actions can be defective.

I will first offer some preliminary considerations and elementary observations surrounding the notions of reason and action.

5.2 On intentions and actions

I will now briefly summarize some of my conclusions from the action-theoretic part of this book. In line with Fulford and most theorists of action, I will presuppose that actions are distinguished from purely bodily movements (and indeed mental 'movements' such as day-dreaming) by being *intentional*. All actions have intentions, although not necessarily conscious intentions. So, if A performs the action F, then A also has the intention to perform F. Indeed, and this is a matter that I shall dwell much upon later, A's intention to perform precisely F, and not some other action, is crucial in identifying his action as the F action. (Thus, in the following, I will exclude the cases referred to in the legal contexts where agents may be liable for acts of negligence, for instance, and thus for actions that they have never intended to perform.) Many contexts exist, however, and to this I will return, where an action is *prima facie* identified as an action of a certain kind by external observers, but where this identification does not coincide with what the agent takes it to be. Such conflicts in identifying an action as an action of a certain type are of course important, not least in a psychiatric context.

For the subsequent discussion, we must also recall the multiplicity of intentions related in a hierarchy. By this, I mean that an agent A, when he or she performs F, need not just have – and typically does not just have – the intention to perform F, but also has an intention to perform G, where G is typically an action lying beyond F; more particularly, in the sense that A believes F-ing to either be a part of G-ing or in some other way be necessary for G-ing. When I intend to take the bus to Kenilworth, I normally do so entertaining some other intention, for instance to have an evening meal. Simultaneously, I believe that I must take the bus to Kenilworth in order to get my meal. (Strictly speaking, I do not have to believe that I *must* take this bus. I need only believe that this is one way of getting the meal. For the sake of simplification, however, I shall restrict myself in the following to the case of necessary conditions.) Now, I may also have some further intention, namely to do some job in Kenilworth later in the evening, and I believe it necessary to have my meal in order to do the job.

I suggest, then, that a hierarchy of intentions is always present – although it may in the limiting case just contain one item – from a highest-order intention, identifying some ultimate action to be performed, to a lowest-level intention, identifying the most basic and most immediate means by which the ultimate action is to be performed. The highest-order action is often of a very general and far-reaching kind, such as getting a PhD or maintaining one's position as head of department. The lowest-order action is what I have already called a basic action.

I would also like to recall the schema for explanations of actions analysed above, called a practical syllogism (*PSI*):

A intends to bring about G

A believes that he is in C

A believes that he will not bring about G in C unless he performs F

A is capable of and unprevented from performing F in C

5.3 On reasons for actions: good reasons, conclusive reasons, defective reasons, no reasons

In the following analysis, my focus will be more on wants than on intentions. In Chapter 4, Section 4.4, I have analysed the notion of a want and pinpointed its relation to the concept of intention. My proposal was that a want is a disposition to form an intention. When A wants to travel to Mumbai, then A is disposed to form the intention to go to Mumbai.

The notion of a want brings us to the topic of reasons for actions. A fact is a reason for action in the light of a want. The fact that it is raining is a reason for my staying home. And this fact functions as a reason of mine because I want to remain warm and dry. I agree with Robert Audi (1993) that this is the fundamental sense of a reason. Strictly speaking, the want is itself not a reason for action. I will, however, for the sake of simplicity of expression, allow myself to make a more liberal use of the term 'reason' in this presentation. I will say that every element in a particular deliberative schema, called *PSW* (Practical Syllogism with Wants), is a reason. Thus, wants come out as reasons for actions and so do certain kinds of beliefs.

Before presenting the *PSW*, I will just say a few words for the purpose of excluding some phenomena from the present discussion. First, I will exclude intentions from being reasons for actions. Reasons are, one can say, not just reasons for actions; they are also reasons for intending to perform the actions in question. Second, a normative mode of speech exists where a person, different from the agent in question, refers to a fact as something's being a reason for the agent to act in a certain way. We may say that the fact that a boy is highly musically talented is a reason for him to enter the academy of music. Here, we are talking about a reason outside the relevant person's mental life. And the implication here is that the boy ought to try to enter the academy of music. This case lies outside the topic of my present discussion. A reason of the above kind becomes *the boy's reason* first at the moment when the boy believes that he has musical talent and also believes that there is a way of developing this talent.

Having left these cases aside, I will now take my starting point in the following *PSW*:

1. *A* wants to bring about *P*

2. *A* believes that he is in situation *S*

3. *A* believes that he must do *F* in *S* in order to bring about *P*

4. *A* believes that he can do *F*

Here, we have no explanatory situation but instead a situation of deliberation. *A* is about to act. He already has some reasons for acting or seeks to find some reasons for acting. 1, 2, 3 and 4, each give him a reason for performing *F*. Together, they give a very good reason for *F*-ing. They do not, however, give him a *conclusive* reason for *F*-ing. This is because *A* may also want to do *non-F* or *A* may believe that it is his duty to do *non-F* (I shall refer to this case as his having a duty-want to do *non-F*). The schema becomes conclusive only when the following clause is added:

5. *A* does not have any reason for abstaining from doing *F*.

I will also say that *A*'s doing *F* is *completely (subjectively) rationalized* if the propositions 1–5 are true of *A*.

Our schema contains what are considered to be typical reasons for action in ordinary life. They seem also to coincide well with what Fulford had in mind in his analysis of delusions. (He exemplifies reasons through the expressions 'this is the way to so-and-so' and 'I want to go so-and-so' (p. 216).) The reasons are then of four kinds. (I shall mostly abstain from referring to item 5.) There is one want-reason and there are three belief-reasons: a belief about an external situation, a belief about means to ends and a belief about one's capacity and opportunity for performing the action in question.

One matter has to be clarified here. Sometimes reasons, even reasons that are obviously a person's reasons, are formulated in terms of an external fact. Consider above the phrase: 'this is the way to do so-and-so'. Or: the fact that it was sunny was a reason for my going out for a walk. These formulations, although very frequent, do not entail any difference – in relation to my above analysis – in the rationalization of an action. It is clear that the fact that it is sunny outside cannot function as a person's reason for acting unless the person is convinced or believes that it is sunny outside.

It is crucial to note that these putative reasons are reasons for a particular action *in the light of each other*. A's beliefs in question are not reasons for doing F unless he also wants to do F (including the case of duty-wants). And the want is no reason for performing the action in question, unless the beliefs are present. So, one can say that citing a reason for an action is citing an element in a set of reasons that are all implicitly there. (Ideally, this set is the complete set entailing reasons 1–5; then we have a conclusive reason for acting.) Thus, a want requires some beliefs (of types 2, 3, and 4) to become a reason for action. And the beliefs of types 2, 3, and 4 require some want to become reasons for action. Moreover, the beliefs require each other.

Wants occur in hierarchies that are completely parallel to the hierarchies of intentions. A want to travel to London, for instance, can in itself be rationalized by a want to meet a close relative (together, of course, with a belief that the relative is staying in London). We may say that John wants to go to London *because* he wants to see his relative. The latter want can in turn have a higher-order reason – say, that John wants to show his affection for his relative. At the top of this hierarchy of wants, we have what I shall call John's *fundamental wants*. By a fundamental want, I mean here a want that is not rationalized by any higher-order want. For example, one's want to survive is one that does not normally have a higher order reason. To say that a fundamental want is not rationalized is not to say that it is uncaused. A fundamental want may very well be caused, for instance by a biological drive. At the bottom of the hierarchy, we have the person's *immediate* wants. Assume that John's performing F is the action to be explained. Then, John's want to perform F is the immediate want of this action.

An interesting field to explore is the nature of the logical relation between wants of different orders. Is it, for instance, the case that John's want to go to London follows logically from the conjunction of his want to see his relative, his belief that the only way to see the relative is by going to London and the fact that he has no want such that he realizes that it is in conflict either with his want to see the relative or his want to go to London? I have elsewhere argued that such a logical relation holds for the case of intentional hierarchies (2000). I am inclined to propose a similar analysis of wants such that this logical relation holds also for want-hierarchies. For my purposes here, I shall, however, only say that in the case where a higher-order want does not issue in a lower-order want (given the relevant belief-premises), there is a great need for an explanation of the matter. (I shall return to this case when I discuss rationality below.)

So much for a basic description of the logic of reason for action. A *PSW*, i.e. a conjunction of reasons of types 1, 2, 3, and 4, constitutes a good (if not conclusive) reason for doing *F*. (After all, even sane people rarely have conclusive reasons for action.) Such a situation of a good (or perfect) rationalization of action will, in the following, be contrasted with one where we say that there is a defective rationalization of action.

5.4 **A note on the concept of belief**

The practical syllogisms *PSI* and *PSW*, as we have seen, make substantial use of the concept of belief, which has itself been left unanalysed. I will not attempt at giving a full analysis of belief here. It is crucial, however, to view 'belief' here as an umbrella term for a number of related cognitive, or partly cognitive, concepts. It is salient that there may be a great variety of cognitive attitudes at play in the determination of action. There is also more than one belief dimension. One dimension deals with strength. The belief can be strong, it can be of the knowledge kind or at least the conviction kind. Or the belief can be weak, it can be of the hint or even the guess kind. Another dimension deals with the relation between the belief and its source. A person's belief can be more or less closely related to his or her perception of the external world. It can be close to or even identical with the experience of an external fact. Or it can be remote from experience and related to it only via information or deductions in the agent's own mind. In the extreme instance, a belief has no link whatsoever to experience. This is the case with the belief in a mathematical truth.

My proviso about the term 'belief' is particularly crucial in the context of psychiatry and delusions. As I will comment on later in Chapter 9, some contemporary theorists (Stephens and Graham 2004, and Gipps and Fulford 2004) have suggested that other cognitive attitudes more adequately called 'understandings' or 'experiences' can occupy the place in the logical schema where I have used the label 'belief'.

5.5 **On various levels of psychological reality of wants and beliefs**

The logic of intentions and wants that I have proposed in this book characterizes in a sense an ideal situation. It characterizes the situation where we have 'real' wants, 'real' intentions and 'real' beliefs. It is of great importance, though not least in the psychiatric context, to consider 'defective' variants of these psychological states. And I am now first referring to defects as to 'reality', not defects as to 'rationality', which will be an important issue below. I wish to identify the 'putative' wants, intentions, and beliefs, i.e. psychological states that may sometimes be confused with wants, intentions, and beliefs.

5.5.1 The issue of consciousness

In all discussions concerning psychological states, the issue of consciousness comes up. The question can be raised whether the 'reality' of wants, intentions, and beliefs, in my sense, has anything to do with consciousness. Must a want, intention, and belief be conscious in order to be real? The answer here is plainly: no. An assumption to the contrary would severely restrict the applicability of this theory. We should not be able even to approach the area discussed by Freud concerning unconscious desires. Moreover, it would be blatantly absurd from a common-sense point of view. Most of our beliefs, wants, and intentions are unconscious in the sense that we are unaware of them. Many such states are unconscious even when they are acted upon. Consider only such actions as are automatized, like driving a car. During the course of a drive, the driver performs a series of rather complicated intentional actions, of which he or she is only aware of a few. But all of these actions are steered by intentions and beliefs. Thus, a lot of actions in fact issue from unconscious psychological states.

To make this observation is not to deny the importance of conscious deliberation for many purposes. It is through conscious deliberation that we can expound the logic of our reasoning and action.

5.5.2 The avowal of wants, intentions, and beliefs

Consciousness is neither a necessary condition of the reality of wants, intentions, and beliefs, nor is it, when present, a guarantee of the reality of the states in question. An agent may be *mistaken* about his wants, intentions, and beliefs. He may delude himself that he intends to do something (perhaps because he is expected to do so), whereas in reality no such disposition on his part exists. We must also notice all *insincere* avowals about one's psychological states. Persons may consciously lie or at least partially misrepresent facts about themselves. Thus, their avowals about their beliefs, intentions, and wants are ultimately not reliable criteria of the presence of these states in their minds.

5.5.3 The question of different degrees of wants and beliefs

A particularly difficult factor, when it comes to the establishment of the presence of psychological states, is that some of them may appear in degrees. This holds at least for wants and beliefs. Intention seems to be more of an all-or-nothing concept.

It is widely recognized that we may have *idle wishes*. These are somewhat like wants. An idle wish involves a pro-attitude towards an object or a fact ('I wish I were married to Sophia Loren'), but a distinguishing feature of the idle wish is that it also contains an awareness of the impossibility of the realization of the wished-for state of affairs. Thus, an idle wish is saliently *not* a want, which is characterized as a disposition to form an intention to act in the wanted direction.

Even apart from the idle wishes, we may recognize various degrees of wants; one can want to have something strongly and less strongly. A natural way of interpreting such degrees is to look at what measures the agent is prepared to take in order to remove obstacles and thus make the realization of the want possible. A person who wants to have something strongly is more prone to acquire this thing than a person who wants it less strongly. (For a more systematic analysis of the notion of a strong want or desire, see Chapter 8, Section 8.6.)

Similar considerations apply to beliefs. One can hold a belief along a scale of conviction. A person has the strongest belief when he or she is *completely convinced*. This is the degree represented by *knowledge* (although the concept of knowledge has a further complexity because of its truth-claim and its requirements as to the nature of evidence). At the other end of the scale, we can conceive of a very faint belief, not much more than a hunch. The complete conviction is certainly sufficient as a basis for action. But so are lesser degrees of conviction. We also have a stage where a belief may be sufficient for a person to take a chance and see if a certain action is conducive to a wanted end or to make an attempt to act in a certain direction, even though the person is not completely sure that he or she can perform the action in question.

For the purposes of this essay, I shall presuppose (when I do not say otherwise) that we are talking about a belief that has the strength of a conviction sufficient to be acted upon, at least in the form of an attempt or a chance-taking.

5.5.4 The property of duration

In order for a want (intention or belief) to become operative, it must of course have some duration. It must at least last until the time of the planned execution. Assume that A wants to get to London before the evening and has found a suitable train that leaves Coventry at 4 o'clock. Assume also that A changes his mind an hour before the time of the train's departure. Thus, A no longer has a reason for taking the train at 4 o'clock. Clearly, he won't take the train (unless he gets a new reason for doing so). Having a want at t for doing F at $t1$ need not result in an F at $t1$. The want must persist until $t1$. Reasons must exist until the time of execution to be operative. (Compare my reasoning about intentions above in Chapter 4.)

5.5.5 **Summing up**

These considerations concern the very existence of a reason for an action to be performed at t. Minimal requirements exist as to duration and psychological firmness for the reason to be a 'real' reason. Already, on this level, we can conceive of defects in a person's mental make-up, which can account for a certain inability to act. Persons may have difficulty in committing themselves and may be inclined to drop their commitments without any obvious counter-reason. However, that a want or a belief is abandoned can in itself be perfectly reasonable. Matters of great urgency may have arisen and may warrant the making of other decisions, or there may be new and more reliable information that may warrant quite different beliefs. Another important thing that may lie behind the abandonment of a reason is that the agents realize that they are not going to make it; they realize that they are unable to perform the relevant action. And belief that one can perform an action is a precondition for one's intending to perform it, which itself is a precondition for the performance of the action.

Chapter 6

On defective rationalization of action

6.1 **Introduction**

So far I have attempted to lay a foundation for the real topic of this part of the essay, namely defective rationalization of action, or the idea of a defective reason for action. I have given an account of intentions and wants and their conceptual relations to actions. I have attempted to show the dispositional nature of wants and intentions and thereby the way in which they can stand in an explanatory relationship to actions. It is important that this explanatory relation may very well be causal in nature. I have also attempted to demonstrate the nature of *rationalization*, which is the particular relation that reasons have to actions in a deliberative situation. I say – with a slight twist of proper speech – that a certain set of wants and beliefs of an agent *A* can rationalize *A*'s acting in a certain way. (What is strictly speaking rationalizing is the content of the wants and beliefs.) Rationalization is a relation totally different from causation. However, the issue can be confused, because the same wants and beliefs as rationalize an action can function (and indeed typically do) as the causes of the same action. In this chapter, let me develop the comparison between rationalization and causation a bit further.

6.1.1 **Acting on a reason: the notion of an operative reason: questions of causality**

I have assumed that wants, beliefs, and intentions can play a part in causal explanations of actions (in the way analysed above). For the sake of convenience, I shall in the following allow myself to say that wants, beliefs, and intentions can be causes of actions, where causes are not interpreted as sufficient conditions but as contributory conditions (or *INUS*-conditions, to speak with Mackie 1974) for actions. This idea has certainly been contested. Luckily, however, much of what I am going to say in the following does not rely on it. The only common platform needed for the following is the acceptance of the distinction between such reasons as are *acted upon*, and such as are not. A man can want to travel to London. Thus he has a reason for travelling there. Still, he may not do it because of a number of preventative factors. Hence, he does not act upon this reason. His want does not become an *operative* want. Another illustrative case is the following. A man *A* wants to visit his aunt in London and he also wants to pay a visit to the British Library. Thus, *A* has two independent reasons for going to London. Eventually, he gets to know that his aunt will not be in London for some months, but he still goes to London to visit the library. In this case his first reason does not become operative, he does not act upon it. It is the want to visit the library which 'makes' him go to London. It is this reason that is effective. In my terminology, the want to visit the library is a (partial) cause of *A*'s going to London.

A set of reasons which does not constitute a good reason for an action, in the sense indicated above, normally does not result in the action in question. (It would, for instance, be pointless for *A* to go to London to see his aunt.) But it is crucial to observe that even good reasons can fail to be efficient. The reason may be inefficient in the sense that even if it indicates a particular action as an appropriate one, there is something which prevents the action from coming about. (I will return to this in more detail below. See Chapter 6, Section 6.2.3.)

In a case where we deal with actions which have already been performed, we can assume that there has been some effective reason operating (if there is a reason at all). This means that if we are going to talk about defective reasons in such a case, we must use 'defective' in some other sense. This brings me to the rational relation between reason and action. I have said before that this is the peculiar relation that the term 'reason' indicates.

6.1.2 Do all actions presuppose reasons?

I will not presuppose that all actions have reasons. I think that actions (i.e. intentional actions) *typically* have reasons and that perhaps almost all interesting actions, excluding now certain actions that may be of psychiatric interest, have reasons. I find it to be obvious, however, that some of our 'little' actions, such as scratching our noses, stretching our legs, even going out for a walk, may lack reasons. Still, they are all intentional actions, although normally not consciously intentional ones. I do not deny that all these action-types *may* have reasons. One may scratch one's nose because it itches and one wants to get rid of that sensation. One may stretch one's leg because it is uncomfortable, and one wants to get rid of that feeling. And obviously, one may go for a walk for a great variety of reasons. My only claim is that such intentional actions exist as lack reasons; in a sense these actions are performed for their own sake. I think it would be dogmatic to assume otherwise.

6.2 **Preliminary interpretations of the notion of a defective reason for action**

6.2.1 **Different senses of a defective reason**

The idea of a defective reason for action can have a number of different interpretations. First, we have the two aforementioned dimensions along which a reason can be defective, namely the causal and the rational. A (set of) reason(s) can be defective in the sense that it is not efficient; it does not result in the action in question. Or it can be defective in the sense that it does not give good reason for the action in question; it does not perfectly rationalize the action. The latter in turn can be interpreted along two main dimensions. First, it may be the case that one or more of the different parts of the *PSW* have some defect as to their rationality. Second, it may be the case that the *PSW* does not itself exhibit any logic. The action in question cannot be 'deduced' from the premises. I will also finally note that the whole deliberation preceding the *PSW* can be defective in various respects.

6.2.2 **The relation between causation and rationalization**

We have already observed that wants and beliefs which do not fulfil the conditions of full 'reality' cannot become operative, i.e. cannot cause an action of the relevant kind. Can they however be viewed as rationalizing it in any reasonable sense? Assume that A (weakly) wants at t to go to London at $t1$ and (weakly) believes that there is such a possibility in the form of taking a train. Does not this reason perfectly rationalize the taking of the train at $t1$? Yes, it does, but I think that it does so under a *tacit proviso*. It rationalizes the taking of the train at $t1$ only under the condition that nothing else comes up that will alter the situation of rationalization. Thus, rationalization is not unconditional until the actual execution of the relevant action.

6.2.3 **Can a set of perfectly rationalizing psychological states fail to cause the action rationalized?**

Assume now that we have a man with a 'real' and sustained want to travel to London on Friday; assume also that he has a 'real' and sustained belief that there is a train leaving his town for London at 4 p.m. and that this is the only train on Friday. Assume also that he has a 'real' sustained belief that he can make it. And assume finally that no conflicting and overriding want or belief exists during the period from the formation of the initial want to the moment of action. Can this set of states fail to result, first, in the forming of an intention to take the 4 o'clock train to London? And can it, second, fail to result in the action of going to London?

Given our definitions of the concepts involved, the first relation must hold. Since we have ruled out that the agent changes his mind, the intention to act must follow from the want to act. The second causal relation, on the other hand, need not hold. This is so for the obvious reason that most actions (the exceptions being certain mental actions and omissions) presuppose a certain physical configuration of the world surrounding the agent. The agent who sets himself to perform a set of actions may fail for physical reasons. He may not be physically capable of successfully performing the actions in question, or he may be directly prevented.

Thus my answer to the question is that a set of wants, beliefs, and intentions which fulfil the reality conditions discussed above and which perfectly rationalize a particular action will invariably lead to an attempt to perform the action in question, and the attempt will succeed if the circumstances are favourable. This is not tantamount to saying that perfect rationalization invariably is causally successful. Even a faint want, and a set of faint beliefs could perfectly rationalize an action but of course not necessarily lead to the performance of the action since the wants and beliefs are so hesitant. The alleged wants and beliefs are not real dispositions to act. The distinction here is important, since rationalization concerns the logical relations between the *contents* of wants, beliefs, and intentions. Causation in its turn puts demands on the psychological strength and endurance of the psychological states of wants, beliefs, and intentions.

6.3 Defective parts of a *PSW*: the case of defective beliefs

Beliefs can be defective in many senses. Some of these must be excluded from the present discussion. A belief may perhaps be *immoral* or *forbidden* for religious, political, or other conventional reasons. If one believes that Jesus Christ was gay one may hold not only a false belief but also a forbidden belief. If, in the Soviet Union before 1990, one believed that a communist state could have defects, then one possessed a belief which was politically forbidden. This kind of defect will not be considered here. (There may be interesting psychiatric interpretations, though, with regard to beliefs which touch the taboo.)

Instead here I will concentrate on such properties of a belief as may warrant the label 'irrational' for the belief in question. Here I distinguish a number of cases.

6.3.1 Incoherent beliefs

A person who believes that both p and $non\text{-}p$ hold at the same time has an incoherent belief. A logician would say that such a belief is irrational and logically forbidden. An interesting problem is whether such a belief is even psychologically possible. The fact that somebody may claim that he or she holds both *p* and *non-p* is not tantamount to saying that he or she actually believes this conjunction to be true. It is probably true that it is psychologically impossible to combine the insight – and I now mean the real insight – that something is a contradiction and at the same time believe it to be true. However, it is very easy to imagine that a person holds a conjunction of propositions to be true and it then turns out that this conjunction is as a matter of logical fact contradictory. (For an interesting analysis of apparently contradictory beliefs in self-deception, see Gardner 1993.) Thus I conclude that it is psychologically possible to entertain a contradiction in this latter sense. This is my first interpretation of an irrational belief (the coherence sense).

But can such a belief function at all in the rationalization of an action? Consider the following case. Liza who is a registrar in a hospital has received a patient. The patient has been in an accident and as a result had an internal bleeding of a particular kind. This bleeding can be the sign of a particular illness which receives a certain coding in the system of registration of patients. There is a clause in the regulations, however, which says that the bleeding should not be classified as this illness when it has been caused by an accident. It should then be registered in the column of accidents. The registrar knows all about this but neglects it, perhaps because of fatigue, when she receives the patient. She classifies the bleeding as *both* an illness and an accident. She does so, on the belief that the patient has both an illness and an injury caused by an accident. This is an inconsistency according to the system of definitions, which she is indeed deep down aware of. However, this inconsistent belief can rationalize (and internally perhaps even perfectly rationalize) the performance of an action described as: registering the patient as having an illness of type *T* and having an injury of type *I*.

This case can be problematized from at least two points of view. The first argument says that the action of classifying somebody as both ill and injured is a non-action. The system of actions is in this case conventionally defined and, according to the constitutive rules for the actions in question, no such thing can exist as registering the patient as both ill and injured. As soon as the mistake is discovered the registration will be annulled and something else be inserted instead. The argument, then, is that no action whatsoever has been performed. Thus the inconsistent belief has not functioned as a reason for any action.

I do not think that this argument holds. It may be true that one cannot say that the registrar has performed the action of classifying the patient as both ill and injured, but this does not mean that she has not done anything at all. She has performed an action that *she has taken to be* classifying the patient as both ill and injured. And she has performed the collateral action of entering two diagnoses in two different columns. Thus a level of description exists on which the registrar has performed a completely possible action.

The other argument would say that what I have just described is not one but two actions. The situation should then according to this argument be analysed as follows. One part of the inconsistent belief rationalizes one of the two actions, namely the classification of the patient as ill. The other part, the contradictory part, rationalizes the second action, namely the classification of the patient as injured. Under this interpretation one cannot say that the inconsistent belief rationalizes any common action, but two different actions.

In conclusion I would say, then, that a contradiction that is recognized by the subject cannot rationalize an action. However, an unrecognized contradiction can rationalize an action. The contradiction (as a contradiction) does not, then, appear among the reasons.

6.3.2 **Illogical reasoning**

I noted above that it is psychologically possible to entertain a conjunction of propositions: p and $non\text{-}p$, and hold the conjuncts to be true as long as one does not 'see' the contradiction. Indeed, if the propositions are complex most people could fail to immediately classify the conjunction as a contradiction. We can make similar observations with regard to reasoning.

Chapman and Chapman (1973) have made extensive investigations comparing normal adults and people with diagnosed schizophrenia with regard to logical reasoning. The hypothesis was that there would be a significant difference between the normal group and the group of schizophrenics in this respect. One of the syllogisms tested had the following form:

All A are B

Some C are B

The question put to the people participating in the test was: what conclusion can be drawn from these two premises? It appeared that in an average group of college students 75% drew the invalid conclusion that some C are A. The frequency of invalid conclusions was not higher among people with the diagnosis schizophrenia.

Thus rationality in the sense of an ability to perform valid logical reasoning (outside the most obvious cases) is not significant for normal adults.

6.3.3 **False beliefs**

One common interpretation of the notion of irrational beliefs (including the psychiatric context) is simply the one that the belief is false. I would argue, however, that it is unreasonable to say that false beliefs, just because of their falsity, are irrational. This contention is not founded on any deep metaphysical theory of truth or a theory which rejects the notion of truth. My whole analysis will be pursued on the basis of the naive idea of truth as correspondence with facts. The reason why this interpretation is unreasonable is simply that we are all – even the most insightful among us – holding a great many false beliefs at every moment. Perhaps most of our beliefs are in the ultimate analysis false. Thus, labelling all beliefs, which may eventually turn out to be false, as irrational does not fulfil a reasonable purpose.

Probably the person who calls a false belief irrational implicitly presupposes something more, in fact intending that it is only a subset of false beliefs which qualifies as irrational. Let me as an illustration quote a traditional characterization of the concept of delusion: 'A delusion is a false belief, firmly held by the patient, which is not consistent with the information available to him and the beliefs of his cultural group, and which cannot be dispelled by argument or proof to the contrary' (Leff and Isaacs 1990, p. 50). Here is a strong requirement. A requirement of inconsistency exists, although this is not necessarily of the strong kind discussed above. We need not have any inconsistency of beliefs, but only an inconsistency between a belief and the information available and between the patient's belief and most other people's beliefs in the cultural group. The requirement of stubbornness in the face of contrary evidence is also present in this case.

I will trace the various subcategories of false beliefs which appear here.

1. *Cultural irrationality.* A person has a false belief which is not consistent with firm beliefs held in his or her society. This is indeed an important interpretation of which there are many illustrative examples in the history of ideas. It has, however, to be qualified. Not all such beliefs have been labelled as insane. First of all, the belief itself must concern a matter of some dignity, such as the existence of god, the fundamental nature of the universe, the value of a political ideology, or the validity of a scientific method. Second, although many people have been persecuted for holding such 'false' beliefs they have often been persecuted because of their being a threat to society, not necessarily because their beliefs are a sign of irrationality or even illness. However, there are indeed cases in history where a person's beliefs have been considered to be sufficient evidence of his or her mental illness. Prominent examples were all the explicit non-Marxists in the former Soviet Union who were taken into custody diagnosed as schizophrenics.

We have a problem, though, with the conjunction 'false belief which is in conflict with a central common belief in the society'. One can easily show in retrospect that many of the classical persecuted beliefs were as a matter of fact not false (and, indeed, that the common 'legitimate' belief has been shown to be false). Thus the interpretation must be 'a belief that is *believed to be false* and in conflict etc.' Moreover, 'falsity' must not here be interpreted in a limited philosophical sense. Philosophers do not normally talk about 'false' values. Perhaps we should instead suggest the label 'valid' to cover the relevant field here.

2. *Evidence-resistant irrationality.* A factor which has often been cited in the psychiatric texts (like the one above) is the person's immunity to such evidence as tends to support the contrary of his or her belief. A boy who firmly believes that he sees a snake in front of him is confronted by his family with overwhelming evidence that the object in question cannot be a snake. For instance, the object does not move, in spite of provocation; it has the wrong colours; it is of the wrong size, etc. Nevertheless, the boy maintains that the object is a snake. We then have a situation of incomprehensibility. The boy does not respond 'rationally' to ordinary evidence and he cannot himself provide an acceptable piece of evidence. He obviously has a deviant concept of evidence, one which appears incomprehensible to outsiders.

This consideration is crucial. The clause about falsity comes out as completely redundant. The reason why we want to attribute some defect to the boy is not that he has (what we consider to be) a false or invalid belief. The reason is instead that he completely disregards what we take to be good evidence and that he cannot persuade us that he has a different piece of good evidence for his case. Thus we can introduce the following main sense of irrationality.

6.3.4 Unjustified beliefs

The boy, then, has what we call an *unjustified belief*. To this I will add: the sense at issue here is that of objectively (or intersubjectively) unjustified beliefs. The boy may very well have a subjective justification. He may be convinced that his belief is completely justified and he may even be able to formulate his rules of inference. We can, however, certainly also conceive of cases where there is even a lack of subjective justification. Two cases can be discerned. First, there is a lack of justification because the question does not arise in the boy's mind. He does not think that he needs justification. He is still completely convinced in his belief. According to the second interpretation the boy is aware that his belief lacks justification. Nevertheless, *he cannot help believing* what he does.

I believe that only a limited set of intersubjectively unjustified beliefs (which also exist in the face of clear evidence to the contrary) can be relevant for the judgment of mental illness or disorder. (I am now not just talking normatively but descriptively, in accordance with what I believe to be the practice.) All people have a range of such unjustified beliefs about many little things. I myself have several unjustified beliefs about other people's characters, about the geographical location of places, about the powers of certain drugs, about the weather tomorrow, etc. I persist in these beliefs although I deep down may feel that they are unwarranted. The reason why I do so may vary from laziness to a wish to have a certain picture of the world in order to retain my peace of mind. I may be afraid that I would become quite disturbed and unhappy if I had to face the fact that Mr. A turns out to have a good character, or that Rome and New York are on the same latitude, or that my favourite pill does not contain any substance which is efficient at all with regard to my present symptoms. The reason why I have not yet been put into custody is possibly the following. So far my unjustified beliefs have not considerably impaired communication with my fellow human beings, and these beliefs have not prevented me from being a functioning member of the society. Nor have I become deeply depressed or disabled. Another important factor is probably the following. If there were to be a confrontation concerning my rational ability on this point, for instance if it was proved to me that Mr. A had in actual fact devoted his life to a good cause, or if I was shown an authorized map demonstrating the situation of Rome and New York and was given a lesson about my favourite pill, then I would probably, although reluctantly and not happily, concede that I had been wrong on these points. I probably deep down share a philosophy of evidence with my fellow human beings, at least on a common-sense level.

Thus, the idea of an (intersubjectively) unjustified belief has to be qualified (as a criterion of mental disorder). *The unjustified belief must have some significance in the sense that it affects the communicative and/or general ability of its bearer and would be upheld even in the face of overwhelming evidence to the contrary.* A special subspecies of such an unjustified belief which is of particular interest for psychiatry is that where the mentally disordered subject has, as we say, no insight into his or her illness. For schizophrenia, the lack of such insight is indeed a typical sign of the occurrence of the illness in question. (For a discussion, see Amador and Kronengold 2004.) I will return to more general characterizations of mental disorder in Chapter 7.

6.4 On defective wants: the idea of an irrational want

It is fairly straightforward to interpret the idea of an irrational belief, in terms of logic and in terms of empirical evidence, as I have just done. But what could it mean to have an irrational want?

6.4.1 **The idea of an illogical want-structure**

There is first one simple logical interpretation. Assume that A wants to have P. A also believes that having Q is a necessary condition for getting P. Then, presumably, A must also want to have Q (given that he or she has no independent reason for wanting to reject Q). If a particular person does not in fact want Q in such a situation, then he or she is irrational.

As I have already noted, it is hard to see that this is a possible case. (For a more formal discussion concerning this, see Nordenfelt 1974.) The most plausible interpretations of this kind of situation are the following: Either A does not 'really' want P, i.e. just claims to want P and perhaps just has an idle wish for P, or A (insincerely or mistakenly) just claims not to want Q. Strictly speaking, then, it is not the conjunction of the want for P and the lack of want for Q that is irrational (if the definitions are correct this is an impossible case); it is the *claim* concerning this conjunction which is irrational.

6.4.2 **The idea of an unrealistic want**

A person may have an 'insanely' unrealistic want. Assume that a girl with an ordinary talent for the high jump wants to become the Olympic champion in this branch of athletics. Her nearest and dearest tell her that she is completely unrealistic about this, but she is not affected. She starts training hard but does not obtain results that are anywhere near an elite level. She is not disturbed by this fact and persists in her ambition.

In analysing this case we must assume that the nearest and dearest are clearly right in their judgment. There are of course interesting cases when a person with an 'unrealistically' high ambition has in fact succeeded. I will here only consider the blatantly unrealistic case.

This case seems in the last analysis to be parallel to the case of incoherent beliefs. There is a lack of logic in the belief structure. The girl already knows a number of relevant things concerning her sport. She knows that the elite athletes jump almost 2 metres whereas she is well below 1.50. She knows what her training has led to so far. She knows a lot about the achievements of her mates and how much they put in with regard to training, etc. In a way she knows, or ought to be able to deduce, that she will not be able to reach her goal. Nevertheless, she believes that she will be able to win an Olympic gold medal. At least this is shown as soon as she starts acting on her want. When a person starts acting he or she has decided or otherwise formed an intention to act. And, according to our definitions, when A intends to achieve P, then A believes that A can achieve P. So, in the limiting case we have here: A believes that A can achieve P, and A believes that A cannot achieve P, i.e. it is a case of incoherent beliefs.

However, one might find intermediate cases where there is no blatant inconsistency. I suggest the following. *A* wants to win the Olympic high jump. *A* acknowledges that *A* cannot realize this. However, *A* starts training as if he or she were training for the Olympics. *A* has then formed some intention, but not necessarily the intention to win the Olympics. *A*'s intention may be far more modest, for instance, to jump higher than the local athletes or to explore his or her own limits in the high jump.

The case of an unrealistic want can then often be analysed in terms of irrationality of beliefs, in the sense envisaged above. The irrationality does not lie in the want but in the set of beliefs supporting the want.

6.4.3 **The case of wants that are out of character**

Assume that a man has all his adult life worked for the Red Cross and for the support of the poor in the Third World. He has been a member of the Red Cross for many years and has never shown any other political interest. Suddenly it appears that this man has during the past month repeatedly steered funds intended for the Red Cross to the support of the anarchist party in his country. Given his previous devotion to the purposes of the Red Cross, the latter acts can be considered as completely out of character. They seem irrational in a sense different from the aforementioned ones.

The situation can be interpreted in different ways. One analysis is that the man has genuinely changed his mind. He may have got disappointed with the Red Cross; he may consider their work futile. He may think that it is no longer meaningful to work within such an organization. If one wants radical political change, then other measures are necessary, he may think. Under this interpretation we cannot sensibly talk of irrationality. The person has undergone a genuine and (at least relatively) permanent change of outlook which, we may assume, is sustained by reasoned beliefs.

Another natural interpretation is that the man has for a long time in fact had *conflicting* wants. But the conflicts have always in the past been resolved in favour of the Red Cross. Perhaps something has happened now which has moved the balance towards the anarchist party. There may be either more or less trivial explanations of this. The man may have fallen in love with an anarchist woman. Or he may have become disappointed with the Red Cross just sufficiently for taking this radical step. Thus, under this interpretation there has all the time been a conflict where the balance has now moved. This is no case of irrationality.

But does an interpretation of this case exist where the want can be labelled irrational? Consider the following situation. The man has not genuinely changed his mind. He does not really know anything about the anarchists, even less does he genuinely sympathize with their ideas. Nor has there been a conflict going on for some time. No woman or any other important external factor can easily explain the man's latest actions. In short, no obvious rationalization exists at all. Perhaps the man cannot himself offer an explicit rationalization. He has on the surface steered the money *for no reason at all* to the anarchist party. (I will return to this below as a case of *arationality*.)

Another alternative is that he presents a belief which is completely unfounded. He may offer as a reason for his action a belief about the anarchist party – for instance that it is much more effective in the assistance of people in the Third World – which, we assume, is totally unfounded. We then come down again to a case of irrational beliefs.

6.4.4 Irrational wants in the sense of self-destructive wants

So far I have analysed irrational wants completely in terms of the irrational beliefs which explain them. However, can we not find any genuinely irrational wants irrespective of beliefs? The only case that I can come up with is that of a *fundamental* want or desire which we want to label irrational. As I have indicated above for the case of intentions, wants can be ordered along a hierarchy from the highest-order, or fundamental, wants to derived wants of various order. The derived wants are all dependent on beliefs concerning the means by which the person can satisfy his or her fundamental wants. The fundamental wants are not dependent on these kinds of beliefs (although they must be dependent on *some* beliefs, for instance about the existence of the kind of entities wanted).

Our fundamental wants tend to be quite abstract. Typical instances are: a want to survive, a want to live a decent life, a want to help one's family as well as one can, or a want to contribute to the philosophy of health. Nothing in principle, however, prohibits a particular want-content from being included in a fundamental want. A want to clean one's teeth, for instance, may be a fundamental want. It is not, however, likely that it in actual fact is. People normally have reasons, in terms of higher-order wants, for cleaning their teeth. Typically they want to keep their teeth in good condition, or they want to avoid the pain and discomfort connected with caries-stricken teeth. However, we probably possess a few quite specific wants which are not motivated by any higher-order wants. These would then also qualify as fundamental wants in my sense.

I wish now to consider fundamental wants of the self-destructive type. A girl A wants to destroy herself, or wants to belittle herself. Again it is important that the wants are fundamental. We can well envisage that A wishes to destroy herself for some higher reason, for instance in order to qualify for a better world than this one after death, or in order to take revenge on her father.

A may even want to kill herself for such higher-order reasons. These cases are excluded here. Assume instead that we have a genuinely fundamental want that is self-destructive. If we call such a want irrational, then the sense is completely different from the ones analysed above in terms of irrational beliefs. The want is called irrational not because it is illogical but because it leads to something that the subject knows is bad for him or herself. To put it concisely: to consciously want a harm for oneself, where this is not wanted for a higher reason, is, then, to have a kind of irrational want. (This analysis is completely in line with the one pursued in Culver and Gert 1982. They define an irrational desire as one involving 'both wanting to suffer some evil and not having an adequate reason for doing so' (p. 35).)

Some may claim that this case can also be analysed in terms of inconsistent beliefs. The logic of this argument is the following. To want P is to value P. If one knows that P is bad for oneself, then one cannot want P. The assumed person believes that P is both good and bad. Thus this is a contradiction and the want must dissolve as soon as the subject realizes the contradiction. My analysis of wants is, however, different. According to my analysis, a want is a certain kind of belief-steered disposition to act. A want can be there without the presence of a positive evaluation of the fact wanted. This also seems to be intuitively quite plausible. An alcoholic may want to have alcohol but he may despise it at the same time. Thus I do not think that the case of fundamental destructive wants needs to be reduced to an irrationality of beliefs.

6.5 A summary of senses of irrational beliefs and wants

In this analysis, I have discerned the following main types of irrational beliefs and wants.

a. *Incoherent beliefs and incoherent reasoning.* A believes both p and *non-p* or A draws an invalid conclusion. These are perhaps the prototypes of irrationality. I concluded that they are psychologically possible at least in the cases where A does not see the contradiction or does not realize the invalidity of the reasoning. I also argued that an incoherent belief can even rationalize an action under a particular description of the action.

b. *Unjustified beliefs.* Having dismissed the idea that all false beliefs should be labelled irrational, I found that there are subsets of false beliefs which have at least historically been characterized as such. First, we have the subset of beliefs which are contrary to (important) beliefs held in society. Second, we have the subset of beliefs which have no justification and are indeed contrary to clear evidence. This is the subset that we normally call unjustified beliefs. Here, we may distinguish between the *objectively* unjustified belief which is a very common case, and the *subjectively* unjustified belief, which is theoretically more interesting. I distinguished between two subcases: 1. the case where the question of justification is not an issue to the agent and does not come up, 2. the case where the person sincerely believes something, while acknowledging that all evidence goes against this belief. This is a situation which is the most incomprehensible to most of us and it is perhaps the case which is of the greatest interest to psychiatry.

c. *An illogical want-structure.* What I labelled as such was the following case: *A* wants to have *P*, and *A* is convinced that *Q* is necessary for *P*, *A* does not have any reason for rejecting *Q*, and *A* still does not want to have *Q*. I doubted the possibility of this case, given that *A* 'really' wants *P* and is convinced that there is a connection between *P* and *Q*. The plausible interpretations in this area I took to be the following: *A* has only an idle wish for *P*, or *A* insincerely or mistakenly claims either that he wants *P* or that he does not want *Q*.

d. *Unrealistic wants.* Here I distinguished between the cases where a person is *objectively* and *subjectively* highly unrealistic in her ambitions. The former is a common case of irrationality. The latter is more interesting. It entails a person who wants to achieve something nevertheless being convinced that she cannot achieve it. If this person's want issues in an intention, then there is as a result an incoherence of beliefs. The person must then both believe and disbelieve that she can achieve the thing.

e. *Wants which are out of character.* Most cases of wants which are out of character can be explicated as cases involving no irrationality. The case which remains incomprehensible is that where the agent has *no* reason at all for the action which is to be explained. Then, however, there is no part of the set of reasons which is defective. This case becomes one of lack of reasons, to be discussed in the next section.

f. *Self-destructive wants.* I focused here on the case where the self-destructive wants are fundamental, i.e. not rationalized by other wants and beliefs which are not in themselves self-destructive. This is certainly a conceptually possible case and probably also a psychologically possible one. It also represents a type of irrationality which is of psychiatric interest.

6.6 On the notion of defective rationalization of actions, where the parts of the *PSW* are not irrational in any of the senses described

So far I have discussed some important cases where we can talk about defective rationalization of action because some part of a set of reasons is labelled *irrational*.

I shall now turn to the cases where we do not have any irrational parts but where anyway the total set of existing reasons fail to fully rationalize the action in question. I shall start by discussing the case where an action F has already been performed by the agent A. We are then here, in a way, in the *ex post facto* situation and ask: What can it mean to say that there is a defective rationalization of A's actual performing the action F?

6.6.1 The notion of defective rationalization of an action *F* which has already been performed. The lack of a member of the set of reasons

Consider the following example:

1. John wants to have an excellent evening meal
2. John believes that La Bosquet in Kenilworth is the only place in the area which provides excellent evening meals
3. John believes that in the circumstances he must take the bus to Kenilworth in order to get the meal
4. John believes that he is able to take the bus to Kenilworth

The action which he subsequently performs is taking the bus to Kenilworth.

What we have here is a (subjectively) good set of reasons for taking the bus to Kenilworth. Our first interpretation of the notion of defective rationalization is then ready at hand. Defective rationalization can be interpreted as having a set of reasons which is not complete. John has a defective reason for taking the bus if he does not have the full set. Assume that John does not believe that Kenilworth is the place to go to, or that he does not believe that he is able to take the bus, but still does take the bus. Here, then, is a case of defective rationalization in the following sense: *An incomplete set (i.e. a set entailing fewer than four components) of reasons for F is a defective reason for F.*

A first question here is: is this situation understandable? Assume that John does not believe that Kenilworth is the place to go to in order to have a meal. Still he goes there. The simplest and most probable explanation of his action must be that John entertains a different belief about Kenilworth and that this belief fits into *another* good set of reasons. He may want to go birdwatching and he believes that there are some good places for that activity in Kenilworth. His want to have a meal, however, has not yet become 'operative' since he does not know of any good restaurants at all.

So, if John's want to have an evening meal is a defective reason for action, in the rationalizing sense of the word, in the lack of the supplementing beliefs, this is a situation which has nothing to do with irrationality. We all have such defective reasons all the time. We all have a lot of wants which cannot become operative because we do not see any realistic means of realizing them. And we all have a lot of beliefs which have not become operative because they have no place in deliberative schemata of the *PSW* kind.

Let us now change the presuppositions. We assume that John wants to have an evening meal but has no belief concerning Kenilworth's qualities from a gourmet's point of view. Furthermore, he has no other want or belief concerning Kenilworth. For the sake of simplification, assume that he is a foreigner and does not even know of the existence of the town of Kenilworth. Still, on a particular afternoon, John gets on the bus to Kenilworth. Could it not then seem as if he has a defective reason for taking the bus, and that this defect is of a deeper kind?

Here, we can say that no member of a *PSW* for taking the bus to Kenilworth is present. This is the most extreme subcase of interpretation 1. It is a case which prompts a further distinction along an objective-subjective dimension (or better: along an external-internal dimension) in the individuation of actions. We must distinguish between actions as *externally individuated* and *internally individuated*.

When a person gets on the bus to Kenilworth, people would in all ordinary circumstances, preliminarily at least, individuate his or her action as: taking the bus to Kenilworth. The foreigner cannot, however, given the assumptions we have made, individuate the action in this way. Thus he has *no* reason for acting in the way he does, given the standard external individuation of his action.

So, how could the foreigner's action be understood? One plausible explanation exists. He has simply made a *mistake*. The foreigner has mistaken the bus to Kenilworth for the bus to Warwick. Subjectively, then, he is performing a completely different action, namely taking the bus to Warwick. And for the action, thus interpreted, the foreigner may have a very good set of reasons. He may, for instance, believe that he can find an excellent restaurant in Warwick that would suit his tastes. The foreigner's belief may not be objectively well founded. But this belongs to the story described above.

This observation leads us to conclude that if we are going to make any progress in this analysis, we must exclusively consider *the action as subjectively identified*. Otherwise we incorporate all the trivial mistakes into our story. It may certainly be the case that the mistake that has been made is rather grave. The foreigner may have been informed just a minute before he acts about the directions of buses. This may indicate some diminished capacity (for instance of a memory kind) on his part. This is not, however, the incapacity we are seeking in this context.

I will now consider an ordinary Coventry inhabitant who has an incomplete set of reasons for taking the bus to Kenilworth. He wants to have an evening meal.

Some belief is lacking in the rest of his story, though. We can differentiate some cases.

First a case which is still quite trivial. Assume that Coventry-John believes that he is unable to go to Kenilworth. This is the only belief lacking in his *PSW* for taking the Kenilworth bus. He may have broken his leg and may have great difficulty in walking. He fears that he may not be able to move to the relevant bus stop. Thus his set of reasons is not very good. On the other hand, he wishes to try. And *trying* to take the bus to Kenilworth is a slightly different action than taking the bus *simpliciter*. The former clearly does not require the item which concerns the agent's belief about his own capacity. Thus, trying-actions in general have a smaller set of reasons constituting a good reason for acting. Trying to *F*, although different from *F*-ing, may end up in a full-blown *F*-ing. The defect, which we thought we had acknowledged, is in a way not a defect, then, if the process goes via the act of trying to perform the full-blown action.

Consider now a lack of beliefs of the second and the third kind. They are intertwined in the sense that a consideration about means and ends is always a consideration given the situation in which the agent considers that he or she is placed. Can we imagine our agent lacking reason 2 or reason 3 altogether? Lacking reason 2 would involve not making any judgment of one's situation at all. (Observe that here I am not talking about making an 'objectively' reasonable interpretation of one's situation.) It would entail having no perception or cognition of one's situation at all. I think this can only be conceived of in the case of a completely unconscious person. Lacking reason number three is different. One can lack any belief whatsoever concerning means to a relevant end. It is indeed common that one does not know how to go about obtaining what one wants. So we can well imagine John not knowing or believing anything about good restaurants in the area.

So here is an interesting case. John wants to have an evening meal. He certainly has some sense, although rudimentary, of his general situation, but he does not know how to get the meal. So there is in his mind no particular action to be taken in order to get this meal. Still, John performs the action – and he also himself identifies it as such – of taking the bus to Kenilworth. Would this be a paradigm case of a really defective reason for such an action as has already taken place? *The agent has an insufficient set of reasons for an action F, in lacking any identification of what he takes to be the proper means to realize his end, and no competing reason exists which can account for his F-ing.* John wants to have an evening meal but he has no beliefs about means and ends. In spite of this he intentionally takes the bus to Kenilworth and his intention refers to the town of Kenilworth.

This case can be rendered plausible if we presuppose that actions need not have reasons. An intentional action can exist without a previous *PSW*. If I am right our last case can be given a new reading. John performs the intentional action of taking the Kenilworth bus just out of the blue. Any wants and beliefs that he has are irrelevant to this action. These wants and beliefs may be potential reasons for a lot of other actions but they have nothing to do with John's intentionally leaving for Kenilworth. (I admit of course that there is some elementary set of beliefs that one must have just in order to perform a simple intentional action, which must be present also in this case.) Given this interpretation, John's initial want cannot be said to be part of a *PSW* which defectively rationalizes John's going to Kenilworth. The want does not have anything to do with going to Kenilworth at all; most importantly, it does not *subjectively* have anything to do with going to Kenilworth.

6.6.2 **On causal and rational relations between reasons and actions**

The last observation highlights an important issue for the future discussion. If no contact (or no relation whatsoever) exists between a particular want or set of beliefs, on the one hand, and an action on the other hand, it is not sensible to talk about the former being defective reasons for the latter. In order for a defective reason for *F* to occur, *some* relation must exist between the reason and the performance of *F*. And consider again the two plausible relations in this context, namely *a causal relation* and *a rational relation*.

Consider first the role that a causal relation can play here. The case that we shall consider is the one where there is a causal relation between a set of wants and beliefs and an action which has been performed, but where the set of wants and beliefs (although in themselves rational) defectively rationalize the action in question. The cases which come to mind are the ones, often discussed in the philosophical literature, where a causal relation is deviant in that it does not follow the standard route. Consider the following example. A person wants to kill the president of his country. He knows what to do in order to kill him and he is convinced that he can do it. The action that is rationalized here is certainly the killing of the president. But it can very well happen that this set of reasons can cause or partially cause a completely different action. Assume that the potential killer, as a result of his extreme ambition, panics and finds himself unable to realize his intention. He therefore decides to take a tranquillizer in order to regain his usual mood. The action of taking a tranquillizer is then partially caused by the reasons for killing the president. There is a relation between wanting to kill the president and the action of taking a tranquillizer, a causal relation, but the former does not rationalize the latter. So here is a causal relation but no rationalization at all.

The interesting case to consider now is the following. Is there a sense in which we can say that a set of reasons *partially* rationalizes an action – at least as much as we can say that there is some relation between the two, distinct from a simple causal relation – where no defect in the particular parts can be found, but where the rationalization is still not perfect?

We may here again get some help from the distinction between *objective* and *subjective* rationalization. A lot of defects may exist in the objective rationalization. Consider the following type. John may want to have a meal and he believes that there may be some restaurants in a neighbouring village, and he goes there. This is only a partial rationalization, since there may be better restaurants in the vicinity, and John has not considered this possibility. Thus, for an *objective* rationalization to be perfect, the chosen action must be the best choice or even a necessary choice in the light of the reasons.

A perfect *subjective* rationalization only presupposes that the agent *believes* that the chosen action is the best or the necessary choice given his wants and his beliefs about means to ends and about circumstances. The agent may indeed act even if this is strictly not the case. He may choose something, even if he does not believe that this is the perfect choice. This, then, is a case of imperfect rationalization also in the subjective sense.

One may contest whether genuine cases of imperfect subjective rationalization exist. The argument behind this is the following. A woman may very well suspect that the action she chooses to perform is not the perfect one in the circumstances. On the other hand she does not have the time or even the will to consider all possible alternatives. She therefore decides not to check whether there are better ways to achieve the end. Now, *given this decision not to check possible alternatives*, the rationalization automatically becomes subjectively perfect. Given that the agent decides to consider only action *F*, *F becomes necessary in the circumstances* when it comes to realizing the want.

A good point exists in this argument, but here I will not presuppose that this kind of perfect subjective rationalization must always be the case. Instead, I will consider the possibility of rationalization which is even less perfect than in the restaurant example above, also from a subjective point of view.

I will consider the following case: *a.* John wants to have an evening meal; *b.* John believes that he is Queen Victoria; *c.* John believes that he is capable of taking the bus to Kenilworth; *d.* John believes that Queen Victoria, evening meals, and going to Kenilworth have something to do with each other; as a result John decides to take the bus to Kenilworth. Here there is very little objective rationality. But also the subjective rationality seems to have diminished. The reasons do not have the form of a perfect *PSW*. They do not clearly pinpoint a manner of action. Only a vague hint combines Queen Victoria, Meals, and Kenilworth. Still, as a result John decides to travel to Kenilworth.

The only slight element of rationalization here is John's belief that Queen Victoria, meals, and Kenilworth have something to do with each other. But why should we call this a rationalization at all? We have defined rationalization in terms of a syllogism of the *PSW* form. The answer is that we are now considering deficient forms, indeed forms which lack one or more of their components (or some part of a component). What we have in this case is still a want and a belief, part of whose content suggests a possible action in relation to the want.

Here we may also distinguish between two subcases, one which gives more support to the idea of rationalization, and one which gives less support. In the former case, John may entertain the meta-premise: the premises *a–d* are sufficient reasons for me to go to Kenilworth. This means that John is completely convinced that he is behaving rationally. This is the case where John at least believes that his practical reasoning is OK. He is in the deepest subjective sense completely rational. In the second subcase, John lacks such a meta-premise. He performs the action without any confidence that it is a rational action. The question of rationality may not even occur to John. Still, his wants and beliefs function as some kind of operative reason for his taking the bus.

Thus, here I have assumed that, unless there is a causal relation, at least some, however minimal, subjective connection must exist between *A*'s wants and beliefs and a particular action, i.e. a minimal rationalization, for there to be a case of defective rationalization at all. If there is no rationalization the connection can only be a causal one and then we call it a deviantly causal one.

To summarize. It is trivially true that a person may entertain wants and beliefs which have nothing to do with a particular action performed by him or her. This case should not be called a defective rationalization of action, since no connection exists at all between the wants, the beliefs, and the action. The predicate 'defective rationalization' can only be applied to such wants-beliefs and actions as have some connection that is, at least in a diminished sense, rational. Rationalization can be diminished in the sense that the reasons do not objectively indicate the perfect course of action to be taken to reach the wanted goal. Rationalization can also be subjectively diminished in the sense that the person is aware that the course of action chosen may not be the perfect one or the person may know that it is not the perfect one. Rationalization can be imperfect also in the sense that the question of rationality is not an issue to the agent and that he or she never considers whether the action is rational or not.

6.6.3 The notion of a defective reason for performing *F*, when *F* has not yet been performed

I will now briefly consider the case where no outcome exists. *A* has not performed *F*, but we still ascribe to *A* a defective reason for performing *F*.

We thus lack the end-result which was present in the former case and which, at least in several subcases, indicated that there was some causal efficiency (or operative strength) in the defective *PSW* in question. In the present case, we must assume that the defective *PSW* is at least not a sufficient causal condition of the action it (defectively) rationalizes.

We must be clear again about the interpretation of the phrase: 'no *F* is performed by *A*'. We are considering the case from *A*'s point of view. Our interpretation must be: '*A* has not intentionally performed an action which he or she considers to be an *F*'. We must, for instance, dismiss the case where John gets on the bus to Kenilworth believing it to be the bus to Warwick. There, subjectively, John does not perform the action of going to Kenilworth.

I will first consider a trivial case of an inoperative reason. John wants to have an evening meal. He has no idea where to go since he is in a foreign country. His want therefore never becomes operative. He does not perform *F* which would have been natural had he known his way about in the country. This is the natural case of an incomplete *PSW* which because of its incompleteness never results in action. In this sense all of us all the time harbour defective reasons for action. And here is really not a defective reason for a particular action but for action altogether. (This is to be qualified and discussed further on.) We can say that something is a defective reason for a particular *F* only if *F* at all comes into the picture. In the case where no *F* is performed we must therefore assume that John has entertained *the idea of F*. This can be the case if John has a vague idea about, for instance, a restaurant in Kenilworth, and thinks about taking the bus there. He may then, however, dismiss this idea as being too unfounded for him to act upon and he therefore abstains.

The interesting situation of an inoperative reason is the following: A complete *PSW* exists (components 1–4 are present) for *A* with regard to an action *F*. We have ascertained that there is no rival *PSW* accounting for *non-F*. We also know that *A* believes that he or she can do *F* and is unprevented from *F*-ing. Moreover, *A* is not as a matter of fact prevented from *F*-ing. However, *A* does not act upon the *PSW*. We then have a reason which perfectly rationalizes *F* but does not cause *F*. This is indeed an extreme version of the classical *akrasia* (weakness of will) to be discussed below.

Again we may have doubts as to the possibility of this case. From my own point of view, the doubt is conceptually motivated. If a person genuinely wants to do *F*, has no conflicting want to do *non-F*, believes that he or she can do *F*, is capable of and not impeded from doing *F*, then he or she must for conceptual reasons at least try to do *F*. If *A* does not attempt to *F*, then something must be wrong with the premises, this argument says. *A* does not 'really' want to *F*, or has some other 'hidden' want not to *F*, or *A* has doubts about his or her abilities in relation to *F*, or *A* is genuinely prevented from *F*-ing. Thus the conceptual logic of wanting does not permit this case. (The case where some other want conflicts with the basic want will be discussed more fully below.)

However, this conceptual presupposition must not prevent us from analysing some slight deviations from the presented case which are 'conceptually possible'. In fact the situation provides us with the following list of slightly defective *PSWs*:

1. *A* has an idle wish to *F*; *A* does not really want to *F*.

2. *A* has an unconscious want to abstain from *F*-ing; *A* is internally 'impeded' from *F*-ing.

3. *A* doubts whether he or she can perform *F*.

The variations 1 and 3 of unrealized wants occur frequently in all of us. These cases are not odd. We all have wishes now and again which never become full-blown wants (case 1) and we are frequently in doubt concerning our abilities to do the things we want (case 3). Such cases of defective rationalization have nothing to do with mental illness. Nor has case 2, at least not in general. Perhaps, however, interesting subcases exist.

We sometimes experience that we genuinely want to do something and believe that we can do it, but still find ourselves not doing it. We understand that some internal impediment exists but we cannot put our finger on it. Typically, we describe the situation by saying that we do not *dare* to do what we want. We are afraid of something but we are not always able to say what we are afraid of. Some mental disorders are perfect illustrations of this case. I am thinking of the phobias, for instance agoraphobia and claustrophobia. In these cases the object feared is only partially known by the agents. They are afraid of walking in open spaces or of being in a small room, but the higher-order reason for this fear is unknown. Similar fears can be found among schizophrenics.

How should the situation of fear be analysed according to my conception? This question warrants a short digression on the notion of emotion and its relation to intentional action. I will summarize an analysis which I have made in *Action, Ability and Health* (2000).

Consider the following properties of emotions. (i) Emotions are parts of the mind which are distinguished from sensations by not being restricted to any particular part of the human body. One feels pain in one's leg, but one does not feel love in one's leg or any other particular part of the body, such as the heart. (ii) Most emotions are conceptually connected to certain situational facts which are called the *reasons* for the emotions. Some emotions can occur, and this for conceptual reasons, in certain situational surroundings only. A woman can, for instance, be grateful only in the context where she at least believes that some other person has contributed to her welfare or the welfare of someone near to her. (iii) This fact in turn explains why emotions are normally directed to *objects* outside the agent. Consider:

(1) *A* fears the approaching car.

(2) *A* envies the famous film star.

Sensations like 'being in pain' and 'feeling warm' are obviously not directed in this way, nor do they have reasons. The connection between objects of emotions and reasons for emotions can be indicated by the following observations. The approaching car, which is the object of the emotion fear in our example, is also part of the environment which constitutes the reason for *A*'s fear. The film star, the object of *A*'s envy, is that person whose various successes constitute the reason for *A*'s envy.

For my purposes it is crucial to note that many emotions to be found among those which occur in explanatory contexts are also conceptually tied to certain wants (intentions) and beliefs. It is logically impossible to be afraid of a thing *x* if one does not believe that *x* is a threat to one or more of one's most fundamental wants. When a woman *A* is, for instance, afraid of an approaching car, that is so because *A* has a standing want to protect her life and health. If *A* did not have this or a similar want, it would be inadequate to ascribe the emotion of fear to her.

As a summary of these observations about emotions I propose the following partial analysis of the emotion of *fear*: *A* is afraid of *x* only if *A* believes that *x* is, or is part of, a state of affairs (the reason) which is such that it threatens one or more of *A*'s most fundamental wants.

A consequence of this analysis is that when a want is impeded by an emotion it is *eo ipso* impeded by a want which stands in conflict with the original one. This observation brings me to an analysis of the case of conflicting wants.

6.6.4 Irrationality that arises from conflict. On the idea of conflicting wants

The idea that wants may be conflicting has lurked behind much of my reasoning so far. A want results in an action only if it is not countervened by a conflicting want. Let me now analyse this notion and a variety of subcases.

a. *The case where deliberation solves the conflict. No irrationality.* I will first present the easy case. A male scientist wants to travel to London during the weekend to present a paper at a scientific conference. At the same time he wants to spend the weekend with his wife, because it is their silver wedding anniversary this very weekend. The scientist deliberates. He asks himself: 'What are my priorities? Which goal is the more important for me to realize'?

He eventually finds that the anniversary has a much higher position on his scale of preferences and he thus decides to stay at home. His want to stay with his wife results in an intention to do so. The other want is, as we say, overridden.

In this case the mechanism of one want overriding another want is quite straightforward. The agent him- or herself decides. There is a conscious deliberation on the part of the agent.

b. *The case of akrasia.* The classic case of *akrasia*, or weakness of will, is different. Hurley, in *Natural Reasons: Personality and Polity* (1989), characterizes *akrasia* in the following way (p. 160): 'When someone behaves akratically, he is irrational by his own lights; he recognizes what he ought to do, but fails to do it. That is, he is internally inconsistent'. Pears (1984, p. 135) puts it this way: '*Akrasia* is internal irrationality and so it is relative to the agent's factual beliefs and valuations'. Thus in the case of *akrasia*, a deliberation has been performed, or at least an insight exists, which clearly points in favour of a particular action, for instance staying at home, but where an alternative action is in fact performed. How can this situation be analysed in the light of my dispositional analysis of wants and intentions?

First, to know what one ought to do, or to know what action is placed higher on one's scale of preferences, is not the same as deciding to perform this action. The alcoholic who knows that he should abstain from liquor, and still chooses the bottle, need not have decided to abstain. He may just have contemplated the fact intellectually. Thus, no intention is formed. The alcoholic has no ultimate disposition for the right action (which in this case is of the omission type).

But do not cases of 'real' decision (or of the forming of an intention without a decision) exist, where anyway the wrong action is performed? And are they not the 'real' cases of *akrasia*? And do they not contradict my dispositional analysis of wants and intentions? Suppose we have an alcoholic who 'genuinely' decides that he is not going to drink any more. Suppose he follows this decision for a while. He does not touch liquor for a month. Then suddenly, he starts drinking again. Thus we seem to have an obvious case of 'real' *akrasia*. My reply to this is that at the very moment when this man starts drinking, he no longer has an intention to abstain. If the man 'really' performs the action of drinking, then he must have an intention to drink. He must at least for a moment have abandoned his intention to abstain from liquor. And that this can be the case is no mystery. We very often change our minds in similar situations and we understand why.

But can we say that the alcoholic has a deliberation which ends up in a decision to start drinking again? The answer here is partly dependent on our requirements regarding a real deliberation. The full-blown deliberation is in the first place conscious, in the second place reasoned in detail with explicit reference to scales of preference where one possible choice is weighed in relation to another. The alcoholic *may* perform such a deliberation. He may re-evaluate his life and say, for instance: 'I find no point in abstaining from a little pleasure in life. I am not going to live much longer anyway. The important medical considerations in favour of abstention do not hold good for me'. Thus the alcoholic may form a well-reasoned genuine new decision involving a restructuring of his scale of preferences. But it is obvious that when this happens we no longer have a case of *akrasia*. At the moment of decision he no longer thinks that abstention is the thing for him.

I will also allow, of course, for the case of an unconscious decision (or at least an unconscious formation of an intention). Here we approach what we may perhaps consider to be *genuine akrasia*. The alcoholic has once performed a full-blown deliberation resulting in a decision to abstain. He does not consciously repeat this deliberation or engage in any new deliberation. Nevertheless, he starts drinking one night when he is together with his mates. We assume that we are talking about a genuine action on his part. Thus, he must, at least for a very short while before starting drinking, have intended to drink. Most probably, then, a conflicting want has been operating and has 'won' the battle. We can envisage that such a want is of the type: a want to experience the pleasure of intoxication.

I will now pinpoint why we might call this a case of irrationality. The alcoholic's want and intention to drink are irrational not because they have not been carefully and consciously deliberated on but because the alcoholic knowingly intends to do something which in the long run will harm him in a serious way, and he has no other reason strong enough to warrant this self-destruction. This case would then be on a par with the fundamental self-destructive want.

c. *The case of compulsion.* A common conflict is that created by compulsion. This is a conflict which is at least on one level quite different from the previous ones. A person who is compelled to do F typically does not (basically) want to do F, but wants to do something else. But there is a conflict of a sort. It holds between a want to do *non-F* and a conflicting (forced) intention to do F.

Below, in Chapter 8, I will attempt to give a substantial analysis of compulsion. I will here just mention the most essential elements. First, an action performed under compulsion is certainly a rational action. The compelling factor is a reason for a person to do something and it is so in the light of some of the wants and beliefs that the person has. But what makes a reason compelling? My tentative answer (elaborated in Chapter 8 on compulsion) is the following: A reason is compelling when it presupposes, and threatens the realization of, a set of wants (intentions) and beliefs which have become fixated in the agent.

For example, the bank clerk who is threatened at gunpoint is not prepared to relinquish his want to remain alive. It is much more important for him to remain alive than to challenge the robber. The only secure way to remain alive in the situation created by the robber is to abide by his demands and hand over the money.

The general notion of compulsion can become interesting in a deeper analysis of some psychological conflicts. This means that a compelling reason for doing something need not stem from some external event as in the robbery case. We also say that a person can be compelled by *internal* factors. And these cases seem to be of particular interest to psychiatry. In my section on psychiatric examples below I will exemplify from a number of areas – for instance, the compulsion exhibited by a paranoiac, the compulsion inherent in very strong drives, like the sex drive or the drive for drugs (including alcohol), as well as the compulsion involved in cases of obvious brain-lesion.

6.6.5 Irrationality in the process preceding the formation of the *PSW*

My analysis here and above has focused on the *PSW* which (immediately) precedes such actions as the *PSW* is assumed to rationalize and cause. In a sense, then, I am only considering the final stage of a deliberation which may be very long and contain a great number of steps. (This has indeed been indicated when I noted the existence of a hierarchy of wants.) This means that rationality and irrationality can occur at every step in the chain. An agent can, for instance, start an inference from an initial belief that is unfounded and finally come up with a belief which is acted upon. The last belief is unfounded, since the initial belief was unfounded; on the other hand it can be rational in the limited sense that it is the result of a valid deduction. An agent can also start a deliberation with a highly unrealistic want, and through reasoning end up with a particular want which is acted upon. The reasoning may be viewed as irrational since the initial want was unrealistic. However, it may be rational from a purely logical point of view. And the final want which is acted upon may not, viewed in isolation, be unrealistic. A person who wants to win in the Olympic games (an unrealistic want) may at a particular moment from that want derive a want to go out jogging (a highly realistic want).

Another possibility is that a particular *PSW* is not preceded by any deliberation at all. Is this in itself irrational? Here we must distinguish between the cases of conscious and unconscious deliberation. A lack of conscious deliberation is very common. Probably few decisions are preceded by conscious and careful planning and deliberation. Many people rarely deliberate consciously but their actions show a clear and logical pattern of decision-making anyway. A reference to consciousness as a criterion of rationality is therefore not adequate. (This is not to deny that one might design an ideal rational deliberation by setting up criteria for careful conscious planning.) If the unconscious decision-making as a matter of fact leads to the same actions as the decision-making in accordance with the ideal design, then we can fairly confidently assume that the unconscious deliberation is also rational.

But consider instead the case where no deliberation occurs at all, either conscious or unconscious. I have already said that intentional actions exist which need not be preceded by any reasons whatsoever. Should they be labelled irrational? I think that a more suitable term is *arational*. Such actions do not pretend to exhibit any rationality. They fall outside the realm which is under consideration here.

However, actions exist that lack any preceding deliberation, which may be of psychiatric interest. These are the cases where the arational actions become disturbing to the subjects themselves. Consider the man who keeps forming intentions which do not fulfil any further purposes but which in the long run irritate the subject himself and even prevent more important things from being performed. I will return to this kind of case in Chapter 7.

6.6.6 **The case of multiple personalities**

So far I have held one factor constant throughout the discussion. I have presupposed that the irrational subject is one personality, or one self, in the case of whom one can presuppose some coherence of will and thought. However, this need not be the case. The psychiatric literature acknowledges a specific disorder called *multiple personality disorder*. In this disorder the patient can host more than one self, each with its specific characteristics. Reznek (1997, p. 110) describes the condition thus:

> In MPD, a person supposedly develops a number of autonomous selves each with their own personalities and memories, each dissociated from the next. Childhood trauma supposedly forces the child to create autonomous selves to deal with the trauma while the central personality distances herself as a defence. These selves operate in isolation, but may be reintegrated with therapy.

Reznek refers to a famous case that illustrates MPD. An American man, known as the Hillside Strangler, was responsible for abducting, torturing, sexually assaulting, and killing many women. He was excused from his crimes, since the court was convinced his central self was ignorant of the acts.

Radden (1996, see also 2004) has made a deep investigation into the notion of a multiple self. She makes two fruitful distinctions: first, between disunities (i.e. disjoint contemporary selves) and discontinuities (disjoint successive selves); second, between subjectively and publicly disjoint minds. When a person harbours two disunited selves they are operating contemporaneously. Sometimes the subject can be aware of the two selves at the same time. Perhaps an example is when the schizophrenic has the feeling that a thought is inserted into his or her mind. The thought may then have the parallel mind as its source. (Often, though, the subject interprets the phenomenon as a thought coming from outside or from a distinct person.) An example of disjoint selves is the famous story about Dr. Jekyll and Mr. Hyde.

It falls outside this treatise to analyse the phenomenon of multiple personalities. It is clear, however, that this phenomenon has a bearing on our analysis of irrationality. In fact, some of our puzzles above can be 'solved' if we assume the existence of more than one mind. An action may be irrational from the point of view of the *PSW* of mind 1, whereas it may be completely rational from the point of view of the *PSW* of mind 2. Assume now that at a particular moment we (including the subject) have no access to mind 2. Hence the action in question turns out as irrational.

In order to draw conclusions about the responsibility of the 'physical' person harbouring the personalities we must make further assumptions. One could in principle make each mind responsible for its particular doings. In the above-mentioned legal case, however, there is an assumption of a *central* self occupying the place of the person most of the time and mostly to be identified with the 'physical' person. However, sometimes this self is switched off and replaced by a more malignant self, which commits crimes. Hence the central self is not to be blamed. Another complication which can occur is if the two minds constantly interact. Mind 1 may make a cautious deliberation about an action, but when the action is to be executed, the stronger mind 2 annihilates some premise of mind 1 and executes a completely different action.

Gardner (1993), however, argues that the theory of multiple contemporary personalities, which is frequently invoked in order to solve the puzzles of the most spectacular irrationalities, such as the ones in self-deception and akrasia, is a non-starter or at least an unnecessary theory. A summary of his negative argument is the following.

It is commonly claimed (for instance by Davidson 1980) that irrationality involves 'a cause that is not a reason for what it causes'. This thesis, however, does not imply a divided mind, says Gardner. What it does imply is mental distance. Mental distance is entailed by the concept of irrationality: (1) irrationality necessarily involves a cause that is not a reason for what it causes, since if every mental cause were a reason for what it caused there would be no irrationality; (2) given such a cause, an explanation is required for why the mind does not correct the causation, which implies (3) that there are mental states which ought to have corrected the irrational process; which in turn implies (4) that there is mental distance between those states and the irrational cause.

Gardner, then, seems to accept that minds can be split in the sense that different sectors of the mind are disconnected. He rejects, however, the idea that there need be a multiplicity of 'complete' minds.

Chapter 7

Towards a theory of mental disorder: the place of compulsion

7.1 Introduction

So far, I have presented a theory of rationalization in which the concept of complete or perfect rationalization has been spelt out. I have gone on to discuss instances of less than perfect rationalization. In this discussion, I have distinguished between cases in which the defective rationalization is due to a defect in some part of a practical syllogism (*PSW*) and cases in which the defective rationalization is due to some imperfection in the syllogism taken as a whole.

In general, I have tried to shed light on the notion of irrationality of wants, beliefs, and actions. I have noted several senses of such irrationality: in the case of beliefs, incoherent beliefs and unjustified beliefs; and in the case of wants, an illogical want-structure, unrealistic wants, wants that are out of character, and self-destructive wants. I have also distinguished between various cases of holistic irrationality: first, where there is a lack of one or more components in the *PSW*; and second, where the *PSW* is defective in other ways. The latter cases of holistic irrationality include non-specific rationalization, *akrasia*, and action under compulsion.

Although I have so far commented on psychiatric interpretations only in passing, I have already noted that many instances of alleged irrationality (in the various senses) exist that do not warrant psychiatric interpretations. Everybody has his great share of irrationality. Most of us probably entertain some incoherent beliefs, the incoherence of which we have not yet discovered. Almost all of us have beliefs that are objectively unjustified, and some of us have beliefs that are subjectively unjustified, i.e. we have them even in the face of strong (perceived) evidence against them. Some of us can have an illogical want-structure (at least in the weak sense of combining an idle wish and a want that stand in logical conflict with each other). Some of us have unrealistic wants and sometimes also wants that are out of character. A few of us have self-destructive wants.

When it comes to defective holistic rationalization, we find a similar picture. Rationalization can be non-specific in the case of many of our actions. Our reasons often do not perfectly rationalize the specific course of action that we choose. Most of us can be the victims of some sort of *akrasia*. For instance, we can consciously decide to choose a course that we know will in the long run be self-destructive. Many of us can be the victims of an internal compulsion to choose something that we deep down do not want to choose. The irrationality that consists of imperfect deliberation is extremely common. We can still debate whether perfect deliberation ought to always be an ideal for us.

The important question now is: what does defective rationality have to do with the theory of mental health? To this question, we may find several answers. First, a traditional one. Historically, many mental illnesses have been partially characterized in terms of *deviant* behaviour, and this is still common. The understanding of deviancy has varied. One interpretation has been that the behaviour is *immoral*. The deviancy of psychopaths or sociopaths is often characterized as 'impetuous' or 'callous'. Or, 'there is a gross disparity between behaviour and the prevailing social norms' (*ICD 9*, p.195). But another understanding has been that the person is in some sense *irrational*. This is a property that is mainly related to the syndrome of schizophrenia. Here, a typical case is delusion (which was the starting point for this investigation), which among other things means a belief held in spite of strong counter-evidence. Another generic case is what is called disturbance of thinking, i.e. 'thinking becomes vague, elliptical and obscure, and its expression in speech sometimes incomprehensible. Breaks and interpolations in the flow of consecutive thought are frequent ...' (*ICD 9*, p.183). We may also encounter disturbance of volition and emotion. Consider, for instance, 'ambivalence and disturbance of volition' and 'mood may be shallow, capricious or incongruous' (*ICD 9*, p. 183).

On the other hand, as Spitzer, Maher, and Uehlein (1990, p. 231) argue: 'If rationality is equated with logic and certain inductive statistical methods widely used in a scientific context, it turns out that such a rationality is almost useless for the purposes of managing the decisions of everyday life. As everyday life is highly disturbed in psychotics, it follows that there is much more to the distinction of normalcy and pathology than rationality'.

A different answer could be given in terms of a specific theory of health. In present-day philosophy of medicine (as presented in Chapter 3), some competing theories of the nature of health and illness exist. They characterize health and illness somewhat differently, and this has consequences for what are to be counted as diseases. According to the biostatistical theory of health and disease (Boorse 1997), health should be viewed as the absence of disease. Diseases in their turn are defined as statistically subnormal functionings in relation to the survival of the individual or the species. Following this theory, such forms of defective rationalization as those that constitute statistically subnormal functioning should be counted as mental diseases (or illnesses). According to holistic theories of health and illness, on the contrary, illness (or ill health) is constituted by the subject's disability or failure of action (in the absence of obstruction or prevention) (Fulford 1989; Nordenfelt 1995). According to these theories, such forms of defective rationalization that entail, or lead to, the relevant form of disability or failure of action should count as diseases. A further holistic theory, which particularly focuses on disease, is Lawrie Reznek's (1987 and 1997). His definition of disease runs as follows: 'A disease, then, is an abnormal *involuntary* process without an obvious external cause that does harm' (1997, p. 203).

It is of particular interest that an official psychiatric definition of mental disorder exists. I have in mind the definition given in the present *Diagnostic and Statistical Manual of Mental Disorders (DSM IV)*. This definition clearly belongs to the holistic camp. I quote:

> In DSM-IV, each of the mental disorders is conceptualised as a clinically significant behavioural or psychological syndrome or pattern that occurs in an individual and that is associated with present distress (e.g. a painful symptom) or disability (i.e. an impairment in one or more important areas of functioning) or with a significantly increased risk of suffering death, pain, disability, or an important loss of freedom. (1994, p. XII)

Given a general theory of health, like the holistic one, we have at least a rule of thumb for selecting such conditions among defective rationalizations that should have a pathological status. A form of defective rationalization that does not significantly affect a person's choice of life-style or choice of activity should not be considered pathological. The fact that it is deviant (statistically or otherwise) is irrelevant. The fact that it is immoral, according to a prevalent code of ethics, is irrelevant. It should also be noted that some forms of defective rationalization may be deliberately chosen by the subject. People may *choose* to be stupid for fun or as a protest. People may deliberately, at least at times, care little about their lives and live in a destructive or otherwise irrational way. This need not be a sign of pathology. The latter is presumably the case only where *a genuine and enduring disability* in rational thinking and acting occurs. I am then only referring here to the kinds of rationality that are necessary conditions for realizing something important to the subject. This is in line with my own basic analysis of the notion of health, which runs as follows: *A* is completely healthy if, and only if, *A* is in such a bodily and mental state that *A* has the second-order ability to realize all his or her vital goals, given standard or otherwise reasonable circumstances. A key concept here is that of a vital goal. For a thorough discussion of this notion, I refer to Chapter 3, Section 3.1, and my previous texts (1995 and 2000). Here, I will simplify matters and identify a person's set of vital goals with the set of the most important wants that the person has. Thus, when people are unable, for internal reasons and not directly because of some external obstruction, to realize fully their vital goals, then they are ill to some degree.

An important qualification of the idea of defective rationalization as a criterion of pathology, then, is that irrational activity as such is not pathological; it is instead *the inability to be rational in relation to one's vital goals*, in the absence of obstruction or prevention, that is pathological.

7.2 On species of pathological irrationality: the central role of compulsion

An investigation into the various forms of inability of being rational can be taken along two very different paths. On the one hand, one can take as one's starting-point the established list of psychiatric diagnoses and see how these can be mapped on to the possible forms of irrationality that I (and others) have traced. On the other hand, one can consider the various logical forms of irrationality and see which of them obviously do reduce or could possibly reduce a person's general ability to realize his or her vital goals. (The latter project is the one initiated, over the whole area of mental health, by Per-Anders Tengland in *Mental Health: A Philosophical Analysis* 2001.) In this brief presentation, I will do a little bit of both. My exemplifications will then of course be very far from exhaustive.

Before considering the central cases of delusion, I will consider the important set of cases where a conflict appears to occur between two or more of the subject's wants. The subject has, on the one hand, a rational want (in the sense that the want is conducive to further important ends of his or hers). But, on the other hand, he or she also has a conflicting, irrational, perhaps even self-destructive want. The latter tends, in a particular case, to override the former. Moreover, the subject is unable to prevent this situation from occurring. This is, according to my previous analysis, a crucial condition.

A large set of cases exists in which the irrational conflicting want overrides the rational want of a subject because the former is, as we say, of a *compelling or compulsive nature*. I will, in the following, scrutinize this idea, first by analysing further the notion of compulsion and then by considering a number of psychiatric conditions that exemplify compulsion in some sense. It is obvious that the terms 'compulsive' and 'compelling', as used in ordinary discourse, cover slightly different kinds of phenomena.

7.3 On the notion of compulsion and its species: Aristotle, Wertheimer, and Audi

7.3.1 Aristotle on voluntary and non-voluntary actions

I have said that all actions are intended, although not necessarily consciously intended. Thus, the locution 'intentional action' is really a tautology. There is another locution, though, which is sometimes confused with intentional action, but which can be used for important discriminatory purposes. This is 'voluntary action'. Not all actions are voluntary actions, according to the criteria that I have proposed.

In *Nicomachean Ethics*, Aristotle (1934) makes some excellent observations concerning voluntary actions. To him, the voluntary action is one whose origin lies completely in the agent. It should not only be the case that the agent truly wants to perform the action in question. The agent should also know the particular circumstances in which he is acting. Thus, an action may be involuntary for either of two reasons (or both) according to Aristotle. The action may be compulsory, and it may be performed through ignorance.

The term 'compulsory', according to Aristotle, applies to any action 'when its origin is from without, being of such a nature that the agent, who is really passive, contributes nothing to it: for example, when he is carried somewhere by stress of weather, or by people who have him in their power' (*NE Book III*, i, 3).

Here, a distinction must be made between two cases. First, we have the case in which a person is directly carried somewhere without contributing to the movement at all. It is just that the person's body is carried away by some other agent. This is to Aristotle the paradigm case of compulsion. However, according to the theory of action proposed in this book, this is not a case of action at all. What modern theorists of action would call compelled action falls under a slightly different category in Aristotle's philosophy. An example is when a man under threat is compelled to walk to some other place. Here, the man is a real agent, performs an intentional action in walking to the other place – he chooses to submit to the force. He could have refused to do so. Aristotle (*NE III*, i, 10) calls this a mixed case. He suggests the term 'intrinsically involuntary but voluntary in the circumstances' for such actions.

> A somewhat similar case is when cargo is jettisoned in a storm; apart from circumstances, no one voluntarily throws away his property, but to save his own life and that of his shipmates any sane man would do so. Acts of this kind, then, are 'mixed' or composite; but they approximate rather to the voluntary class. (*NE III*, i, 5–6)

Aristotle wishes to emphasize that the origin of the action here is, strictly speaking, within the person himself or herself. It is within the power of the person to perform the action or not. But basically these actions are involuntary. Such an action would never be chosen for itself. It is therefore involuntary, apart from circumstances.

The question can be asked whether the term 'compulsion' or, for that matter, the terms 'mixed' or 'composite', can be applied to acts done for the sake of pleasure or for noble purposes. Or, in other words, is temptation a case of compulsion? Aristotle strongly rejects such a proposition. He thinks that this would make every action compulsory.

> For (1) pleasure and nobility between them supply the motives of all actions whatsoever. Also (2) to act under compulsion and unwillingly is painful, but actions done for their pleasantness or nobility are done with pleasure. And (3) it is absurd to blame external things, instead of blaming ourselves for falling an easy prey to their attractions; or to take the credit of our noble deeds to ourselves, while putting the blame for our disgraceful ones upon the temptations of pleasure. (*NE III*, i, 11–12)

One can wonder why Aristotle is not prepared to accept any kind of temptation as at least a mixed case (involuntary but voluntary under the circumstances). I think one must distinguish between an ordinary action directed towards a pleasant goal, which is indeed the paradigm case of a voluntary action, and such cases where a person is tempted by the prospect of immediate strong pleasure, as in the case of seduction. In the latter case, there is normally some reluctance on the part of the agent. He or she hesitates and is aware that there might be a conflict between what duty prescribes and what yielding to the temptation entails. The issue becomes crucial when we have a case of the so-called 'irresistible temptations'. It could be noted that we sometimes excuse a person for actions performed under irresistible temptation. A pyromaniac who has set fire to a number of houses can be held unaccountable for his or her actions. The reason is that we believe that he or she was incapable of refraining from the actions in question. I will make a case for irresistible temptations in Chapter 8, Section 8.6, as instances of compulsion.

Let me now express the Aristotelian notion of compulsion (strictly speaking, an action that is intrinsically involuntary but voluntary under the circumstances) in a more formal way: A is compelled to perform X if, and only if, A does not want to perform X but still forms the intention to perform X, because not performing X would in the circumstances entail a harm to A that A considers worse than the harm caused by performing X.

What about Aristotle's suggestion that a voluntary action also presupposes knowledge on the part of the agent? First, Aristotle makes the subtle distinction between non-voluntary actions and involuntary actions. The latter is a subset of non-voluntary actions. An involuntary action is a non-voluntary action that causes the agent pain and regret (*NE III*, i, 13). What all non-voluntary actions have in common is that the agent is ignorant of one or more of the circumstances of the action.

A grave kind of ignorance exists, referred to in some celebrated legal cases, where the agent is totally ignorant of what he or she is doing. How is this possible? Can one be ignorant of what one intends to do? (Observe the difference between 'being ignorant of' and 'not being conscious of'. I have already observed that one need not be conscious of one's intentions.) This is difficult to imagine. If one intends to do X, which entails having certain beliefs related to X, then one can hardly believe that one intends to do *non-X*. But, in saying so, we presuppose a coherent personality. Such a presumption cannot perhaps be made in certain psychiatric cases. As Aristotle himself notes: 'Now no one, unless mad, could be ignorant of all these circumstances together' (*NE III*, i, 17).

A more plausible and common case of ignorance is the following. Assume the situation where a woman visits a factory and is curious about the functions of all the buttons that she observes on the control panel in the factory. She presses a button, ignorant of the fact that this button is connected to the closing down of the whole production of the factory. Here, she knows what she does under one description of the action (namely a very low-level description, close to the basic action). But she does not know what she does under the description 'stopping production'. Strictly speaking, she does not, according to our explication, perform the action of stopping production. The breakdown of production is a consequence of her action of pressing the button, not a result of it. The law, however, here uses a wider notion of action. The law has to hold agents responsible for certain consequences of actions that the agents have not themselves intended.

Another instance of not knowing what one does is the following: A man has just joined the Conservative Party and makes a speech using some arguments that he believes to be strong in support of the party. Unfortunately, he is unaware of the fact that these arguments are based on false information and that this has recently become obvious to the public. The consequence of his performance is therefore contrary to his intention. He is in no way supporting this party.

The conceptual tools introduced in Chapter 1, Sections 1.7 and 1.9, can now be applied to analyse the cases of non-voluntary actions. The most extreme case of non-voluntary action is when the agent is unaware of all circumstances of the action, i.e. he or she is unaware of the action under all its descriptions. This is extremely uncommon but may exist among the 'insane'. In other cases, the agent is aware of the nature of his or her action under certain descriptions but not under other descriptions. The agent is typically aware of the action on the basic action level, namely that he or she is moving certain limbs, or on levels close to the basic action, for instance, that he or she is manipulating a physical object close to the body, like pressing a button. The person may, however, be unaware of further possible results or consequences. The woman in our example does not know that she is stopping the production, and the male politician does not know that he is in fact undermining the credibility of his party instead of supporting it.

We can then summarize. Two important subspecies of non-voluntary actions exist, according to Aristotle: compelled actions and certain action-types performed through ignorance. For Aristotle, the strictly compelled action, for instance, when a person is dragged from one place to another, is a non-action according to my terminology. The mixed cases, the actions that are intrinsically involuntary but voluntary in the circumstances, constitute the paradigm cases of compulsion according to a modern terminology.

In my subsequent analysis of compulsion (Chapter 8), I will add some criteria to the Aristotelian account, which I find necessary if the notion is to be applicable to the context of mental disorder.

7.3.2 Wertheimer's theory of coercion

Alan Wertheimer (1987) has presented an extremely well-argued and cautious analysis of the legal notion of coercion. The focus in his analysis rests exclusively on the situation when one human being coerces another to perform an action. This limits the value of his analysis for my purposes, since I have set myself to study the generic notion of compulsion. On the other hand, Wertheimer's analysis contains many reflections that need to be considered by any theorist of compulsion or of similar concepts.

We must first note that Wertheimer's treatise is embedded in a legal context. One half of his book contains analyses of a great number of legal cases where a decision has been made as to whether a person should be considered to have coerced another person. Also, in the purely philosophical analysis, Wertheimer has committed himself to constructing a notion of coercion that is useful for the legal and moral contexts where there is the question of a person's responsibility for his or her actions. His own characterization of the notion of coercion is indeed a moral one. A coercive act is, by definition, an immoral act. If A has the moral right to make B perform a certain action, then it cannot be the case that A coerces B.

However, Wertheimer does not introduce this connection between coercion and morality by *fiat*. He tries very hard, discussing attempts by other authors, to find a non-moral account of coercion that could still do the moral and legal job required to exonerate a person from responsibility for an action. Among other alternatives, Wertheimer studies attempts based on notions of voluntariness and freedom but he does not find any such attempt successful. Let us, then, look at his substantial characterization.

According to Wertheimer, A coerces B to do X only if 'A attempts to get B to do X (which can be a nonaction) in the following way: A proposes that (1) if B does X, A will bring about or allow to happen a certain state of affairs (S), and (2) if B does not do X, A will bring about or allow to happen another state of affairs (T). Coercive proposals are typically biconditions because of the conjunction of (1) and (2)' (p. 202).

Now, this general formula cannot distinguish between threats and offers. In order for a coercive situation to occur, the proposal, according to Wertheimer, must be a threat. The distinction between the two kinds of proposals is made in the following way: '*A threatens B* by proposing to make *B worse off* relative to some baseline; *A makes an offer to B* by proposing to make *B better off* relative to some baseline. More precisely, *A* makes a threat when, if *B* does *not* accept *A*'s proposal, *B* will be worse off than in the relevant baseline position. *A* makes an offer when, if *B* does *not* accept *A*'s proposal, he will be *no* worse off than in the relevant baseline position' (p. 204).

To be able to talk about being better or worse off, one has to define a baseline. Wertheimer shows that there are difficulties involved in deciding the baseline needed. He discusses, in particular, a statistical test and a moral test of *B*'s baseline. To illustrate, Wertheimer uses an example presented by Nozick (1969, p. 449):

> Q is in the water far from shore, nearing the end of his energy, and P comes close by in his boat. Both know there is no other hope of Q's rescue around, and P knows that Q is the soul of honesty and that if Q makes a promise he will keep it. P says to Q "I will take you in my boat and bring you to the shore if and only if you first promise to pay me $ 10,000 within three days of reaching the shore with my aid".

Under the statistical test, the question whether this is a threat or an offer will depend on what is normal in the society. In some societies, it is likely that *A* will rescue *B*, in others it is not. Under the moral test, the question is whether *A* is morally required to rescue *B* or not. If he is, then *A*'s baseline presupposes *A*'s beneficial intervention and *A*'s proposal becomes a threat. If he is not so required, then it is an offer.

Wertheimer himself thinks that the moral test is the only reasonable test '*given* that a coercion claim is meant to have a *particular* moral force such as to bar or mitigate the ascription of responsibility' (p. 212).

Wertheimer, however, also discusses the case where an extremely attractive offer has been presented to *B* and where *B* cannot resist this offer. It is sometimes said that this is a case of coercion. Wertheimer excludes this case from coercion proper. He instead introduces the term 'seduction': '*A* makes a *seductive* offer when *B* is unable to resist *A*'s proposal' (p. 222). Seduction covers the cases where *B* loses self-control, when *B* cannot control some behaviour that he or she prospectively or retrospectively prefers not to engage in, such as drinking, smoking, and overeating.

Here, Wertheimer makes an interesting concession that he does not return to. He says that, even if seduction is not coercive, it might have comparable moral force (p. 224). A person who has been seduced, i.e. been confronted with an irresistible temptation, can be exonerated from responsibility. This concession is crucial to a more general assessment of Wertheimer's theory. Wertheimer's main purpose is to propose a theory of coercion that can function in legal and moral cases. He then excludes certain cases – which are considered in common parlance to be coercive or compelling – from being proper cases of coercion.

Let me now turn to an assessment of Wertheimer's proposal for my own purposes. Although Wertheimer makes a number of sharp and interesting analyses, I fail to see that he can contribute much to the notion of compulsion that is central in mental disorder. Wertheimer does not include in his characterization the element of restriction of freedom or unavoidability that is so crucial to our ordinary understanding of compulsion, not least in the psychiatric context. He is aware of notions of compulsion related to limited freedom, but refuses to accept that they have any bearing on the idea of moral or legal responsibility. (Cf. above, however, his concession with regard to seduction.)

To see this clearly, consider the following example, which fulfils Wertheimer's conditions of a coercive threat: A self-indulgent man tells a young boy Peter that if Peter does not pick up a piece of paper that Peter has dropped on the pavement, then he will tell Peter's mother about it. Here, the man proposes to make Peter worse off according to a baseline. And the man has no right to make this kind of threat; he is not the proprietor of the pavement. Assume now that Peter succumbs to the threat. He seems then to have been coerced according to Wertheimer's conditions.

Assume, however, that Peter does not really mind much about this situation. He does not consider that he is much worse off – although he is clearly somewhat worse off – if his mother gets to know about this incident. His mother would become disturbed but not care that much if an insolent stranger told her about Peter's very minor offence. Peter might very well have shaken the incident off and just have walked away. However, here he chose to succumb to the threat because he found that to be simple enough.

According to Wertheimer's analysis, this is a clear case of coercion. It would hardly, however, be seen as a case of coercion in the sense of Peter being compelled to act. Peter's action is in no way an action that he 'must', or feels that he 'must', perform. There is no element of unavoidability in this case. I think that the notion of compulsion inherent in and typical of mental disorder has this element in it.

7.3.3 Audi's theory of compulsion

I will now consider Robert Audi's modern characterization of compulsion in his influential book *Action, Intention and Reason* (1993). Audi starts his analysis by contrasting acting freely and acting under compulsion. He uses the expression 'could not have done otherwise' to describe the typical core of compulsion. Moreover, Audi discusses the generic concept of compulsion, covering instances where no coercing agent need be involved. Audi says (p. 190): 'Compulsions may be external or internal. The former include such things as blackmail and various threats, most notably that of death; the latter include things like addictions and certain obsessions, phobias and unconscious drives'. Crucial is also that Audi, like Wertheimer and myself, uses the term compulsion only for cases of intentional action.

In order to give a compact and accurate account of Audi's notion of compulsion, which clearly belongs to the Aristotelian tradition, I will use his own summary (pp. 196–197). According to Audi's proposal, the sentence 'A is compelled to F at t' should be given the following analysis:

1. it is not the case that a motive of personal gain is an important part of what motivates A to F.

2. A believes that there is some state of affairs on account of which his or her not F-ing would (might) have very bad consequences.

3. Because of the belief specified in 2, A believes either (or both) (i) that his or her F-ing is so substantially preferable to not F-ing that it would be very unreasonable not to F, or (ii) that, from the point of view of A's own welfare or the welfare of someone (or something) A wants to protect, his or her not F-ing would (might) have the sorts of consequences specified in 2.

4. A strongly wants to avoid not F-ing (or what A believes are the consequences of not doing it), and this want is substantially stronger than any want(s) A may have to avoid F-ing or to avoid any bad consequences that A believes F-ing would (might) have.

5. The beliefs and wants specified in 2–4 constitute at least the main reason why A F-s.

According to Audi, certain non-standard cases of compulsion exist. These include cases where F is not intentional or, if intentional, performed without A having the beliefs specified in 2–4. One example would be one's standing up during a lecture because of a posthypnotic suggestion. A second would be one's being compelled to drink ale because of a sudden overpowering thirst (again, induced from the outside). For these cases, Audi distinguishes the following conditions:

6. Either 1 or, if a motive of personal gain is an important part of what motivates A to F, it is without his or her consent, induced in A by some interference with A's normal functioning, such as hypnosis, implanted electrodes, drugs or surgery.

7. Either 2 or there is some state of affairs that produces in A either simply a powerful (and possibly unconscious) desire to F, or a non-motivational tendency to F in order to realize an extrinsic or intrinsic want.

8. Even if at t (i) A should believe (as he or she may or may not) that F-ing would have a consequence of the sort specified in 2 and (ii) A was as strongly motivated to avoid F-ing as would be appropriate to this belief, A would still F.

9. Either the non-motivational tendency specified in 7, or a set of wants and beliefs of the sort cited in 2–4, or one or more desires of the kinds cited in 6 and 7, constitute at least the main reason as to why A F-s.

To summarize: A is compelled to F at t if, and only if, either 1–5 or 6–9 or both is the case (p. 198).

The crucial element in Audi's standard case of compulsion (1–5) is that no motive of personal gain exists for the subject. To see this, consider the following instance, which is in accordance with Audi's analysis. John observes a young boy who has fallen into the water. John believes that if he does not rescue the boy then a great risk exists that the boy will drown. John considers this to be an extremely bad consequence (condition 2 realized). Saving the boy does not entail any personal gain with regard to John (condition 1 realized). John believes that his saving the boy is so substantially preferable to his not saving him that it would be very unreasonable not to save him (condition 3 realized). John strongly wants to avoid leaving the boy in the water, and this want is substantially stronger than his want to avoid rescuing him. (In the case, we envisage he has no want to avoid rescuing him at all, i.e. condition 4 is realized.) All these beliefs and wants constitute the main reason why John rescues the boy.

The upshot of this example is that any action of duty (where the action does not involve any personal gain) and where the agent believes that the consequences of not following the rule of duty are quite bad (and where conditions 3 and 4 are also realized) is a compelled action. This is a broad notion of compulsion.

On the other hand, it is, according to Audi, conceptually impossible for an agent to be compelled to perform an action that enhances or protects his or her personal prosperity. (Admittedly, Audi is not quite clear here. He refers in condition 3 to the person's welfare, suggesting that the preservation of one's own welfare can be compelled.) An action in order to increase one's fortune (and which does not fulfil the criteria under 6 or 7) cannot be a compelled action. But surely, such egocentric actions occur as we normally consider to be compelled. Assume a financial magnate who has the goal of expanding his empire and that he is prevented by his country's bureaucracy from doing so.

He is then, he thinks, compelled to move to another country that has a more liberal economic philosophy. This is evidently a case where the motive is personal gain. Thus, this cannot qualify as an act of compulsion, according to Audi. However, to me this is a prototype of compelled action. The magnate's act to move abroad is an action that he is, given his intentions, forced to perform. The actions of the authorities in his own country threaten his financial ambitions.

It seems to me, then, that Audi, in his characterization of the standard case of compulsion 1–5, does not capture the element of unavoidability or 'not being able to do otherwise' that he himself finds essential when he initiates his analysis. However, by introducing the non-standard form of compulsion 6–9 Audi notes some crucial cases of unavoidability, namely the cases of desires induced by the use of drugs or the experience of overwhelming events. It is important to analyse these cases, not least in the psychiatric context. On the other hand, they do not cover the essential instances of compulsion in ordinary contexts where there is an element of unavoidability. My examples above indicate these. This notion of unavoidability does not exclude the idea of a personal gain. One can be compelled to perform actions that may or may not lead to personal gain.

Audi seems to be partially aware of this fact in his further discussion of moral responsibility. He observes that compulsion cannot be sufficient for exoneration from responsibility. Therefore, he adds some conditions to his account of compulsion in order to approach the idea of unavoidability that is present in our ordinary thinking on compulsion. He says that A could not have acted different from what he did if, and only if, A was compelled to do F and he could not reasonably be expected to have avoided doing F or no morally sound person could reasonably be expected to have done otherwise (p. 202). Apart from the fact that I think that compulsion already contains the element of unavoidability, I find this supplement still insufficient to capture the notion of unavoidability. (See my own characterization in Chapter 8.)

We may recall that compulsion has, in much traditional legal thinking, been confused with such a strong notion of unavoidability as complete determination (see the following chapter). According to the thinkers in this tradition, a compelled action is one that has been sufficiently conditioned by a set of internal events. This kind of determination does not distinguish between actions that do or do not involve personal gain.

I think 'unavoidable' actions in some sense exist, and that they may lie in one's self-interest (and not be induced by drugs, etc.). I think that actions exist that are strongly motivated by duties (where the subject considers the consequences of not fulfilling the duty to be very bad) that are not unavoidable. This sets the stage for my own analysis.

Chapter 8

Towards a new analysis of compulsion

8.1 **Introduction**

According to the analysis of compulsion that I wish to endorse and which I think is relevant in a psychiatric context, compulsion has to do with unavoidability. The person who is compelled could not – in a certain sense – have acted otherwise than he or she did. Consider:

(i) *A* was compelled to do *F* at *t* if, and only if, *A* could not avoid doing *F* at *t*.

A first interpretation of this locution is that *A*'s doing *F* is strictly determined. According to this idea we could conclude from a complete description of the world at time *t*, together with a statement of the relevant general laws, that *A* would perform *F* at *t1*. It is important to realize that this deterministic interpretation of compulsion has had a place in the history of ideas. It has been particularly prevalent in forensic psychiatry, where the alleged existence of deterministic compulsion has been used as an argument for the abolition of punishment in the case of certain mentally ill offenders. (I have discussed this at length in the Swedish forensic context in Nordenfelt 1992 and 2000.) The argument runs as follows. A mentally ill offender may have committed a crime under internal compulsion. A compelled act is an act which has been strictly determined, i.e. sufficiently caused by internal or external events. Sufficient causation excludes the possibility of free will. Free will is necessary for responsibility. Thus people cannot be responsible for such doings of theirs as have been sufficiently caused.

Determinist critics of this view have maintained that all actions must be sufficiently determined. Therefore, all agents are completely determined in all their actions. Hence the notion of responsibility turns out to be useless for the differentiation of compelled and non-compelled actions. (See, for instance, Menninger 1968.)

I wish to argue that this interpretation of compulsion is unreasonable when it comes to (most cases of) what is commonly called compulsion in both ordinary and psychiatric contexts. Note that here I am not trying to defend a particular metaphysical thesis about causation of action or about free will. For all we know, determinism may, in spite of the present state of the theory of physics, be true. But if determinism is true then both the so-called compelled actions and uncompelled actions are equally sufficiently determined by their initial conditions. In that case there is no point in trying to single out compelled actions from other actions. As long as we find it reasonable to distinguish certain actions that we cannot, as we say, avoid performing, from other actions that we can avoid performing, then we must find some other criterion for differentiating between the two. The notion of compulsion is, I think, a fruitful, indeed a necessary, one in many ordinary-life contexts as well as in psychiatry. I will therefore introduce quite a different analysis of it.

Consider first compulsion in an explanatory context. The statement 'The soldier shot at the enemy because he was forced to do so' is a reasonable action-explanation. The fact that an agent is compelled or forced to perform a certain action is sometimes cited as the explanation of the action. This case is, I shall claim, a subspecies of rational explanation (see above Chapter 4, Section 4.5.2).

On the surface of it this kind of explanation is far from rational or even intentional explanation. A person who is forced is said to have 'no choice'. I will, however, here challenge this *prima facie* impression. A compulsion or a force is instead a reason (normally external) for an agent to perform a certain action. This may be brought out in the following analysis. *A* is a private in the Swedish army during wartime. *A* is ordered by his officer to shoot at an enemy platoon approaching his position. *A* knows that if he does not shoot, he will be court-martialled and in the end be sentenced to death. *A*, however, intends to survive. Hence he will shoot at the enemy.

This case is in all essentials on a par with the example of an approaching car that makes a person jump away. The only slight difference lies in the surface locutions. In the case of the approaching car the reason is spelt out in detail. In the force-case, the locution can sometimes be quite elliptic: 'He acted because he was forced to do so'.

In this chapter, I will go deeper into the analysis of the notion of compulsion in an action-theoretic context. This analysis will be quite general and not tied simply to an ethical or legal context. In several previous analyses, the concept of compulsion has been analysed solely with regard to the case where compulsion is a justification of or excuse for moral or legal wrongdoing. (See my discussion of Wertheimer's theory, Chapter 7, Section 7.3.2.) This is a crucial situation but it is not the only possible one. The context of mental illness, which is my own focus of interest, is another crucial context.

My analysis will also question the naive assumption that compulsion is an all-or-nothing matter, i.e. the idea that you are either compelled to do something or you are not compelled to do it. My proposal involves the suggestion that several degrees of compulsion exist, from total compulsion to a low degree of compulsion. Given the idea that compulsion and the feeling of compulsion are central ingredients of mental illness, the assumption of degrees of compulsion can be reflected in degrees of mental illness.

The action-theoretic framework must be observed. Compulsion here concerns human intentional action. A person who is dragged from one place to another is not compelled in my sense. Being dragged is not to perform any action at all. It is to be the object of *physical force* (see below). Thus compulsion must go via the compelled person's intentions and beliefs. When A is compelled to do F, it must still be practically possible for A to perform *non-F*. However, in the light of A's intentions and beliefs, F is for A the only thing to do. Thus the initial formula (i) must be rectified:

(ii) A was compelled to do F if, and only if, A could not avoid doing F in the light of A's intentions and beliefs.

Compulsion is often but not necessarily an interactive concept in the following sense: Agent A (the primary agent) acts towards agent B (the secondary agent) in a way such that B is compelled to perform F. This interactive case of compulsion is often called *coercion*. Only human beings can coerce other human beings. However, natural events and states of affairs can compel people to act. I will in a later part of this chapter discuss the general case that also covers the compulsion executed by natural states and events. (For a different use of the term 'coercion', see Watson, 1977.)

8.2 A starting-point: the practical syllogisms

In order to initiate my analysis, I will present the context of deliberation:

A wants to bring about P

A considers that A is in C

A considers that in C A's doing F is one of A's possible actions to bring about P

A can do F

In the context of deliberation, A considers several possible actions to bring about P in order to settle on the most efficient or, in general, the best one. It is essential to a situation of deliberation that alternatives exist and even that the want can be changed, at least in the sense that it can become modified during the process of deliberation.

Assume that George wishes to travel from Linköping to Stockholm on Friday evening. George consults the timetables and also reflects on his own needs and preferences with regard to the arrival. He concludes that it is desirable to reach Stockholm before 7 o'clock and that the most convenient way to reach Stockholm before that time is to take the 5 o'clock train which reaches Stockholm a few minutes before 7. As a result of this deliberation George decides to take this train, and his intentional practical syllogism can be given the following form:

George intends to reach Stockholm just before 7 o'clock on that Friday evening

George is convinced that given that he starts from Linköping a certain set of possible means of communication exists

George is convinced that in order to reach Stockholm just before 7 o'clock on that Friday evening he must take the 5 o'clock train from Linköping

George can take the 5 o'clock train

The schema of deliberation has thus become transformed into a syllogism (*PSI*) issuing in George's taking the 5 o'clock train. The intentional version of the syllogism presents no alternative. Given the premises (and given my analysis of these premises, discussed in Chapter 4, Section 4.3), it follows logically that *A* does *F*. According to this analysis of the syllogism, it is a binding logical conclusion. In a sense (the weakest sense, which is to be qualified later), the agent *A* is here compelled to perform *F*.

It is counterintuitive, however, to call this situation a situation of compulsion in the ordinary sense of the word. If this were a case of compulsion, then all actions would be compelled. Since every intentional action can ultimately be viewed as issuing from such a practical syllogism, then every intentional action would become compelled. The distinction between voluntary and non-voluntary (i.e. compelled) actions would then fall apart. We would have no use for the notion of compulsion.

But why does the syllogism not capture our intuitive sense of compulsion? The reason is that the premises in the syllogism are (normally) not, as I would say, *fixated* in the sense that they cannot be altered. The premises can (normally) be changed either by the agent's will or by the course of events. A person may abandon an intention by will; he or she may arrive at new conclusions with regard to the circumstances at hand or with regard to the means necessary for attaining the intended end. Finally, a person may lose the capacity or opportunity for performing the action.

The standard case of action determination becomes a case of compulsion, I suggest, when the premises are *fixated*, i.e. when the premises are not changeable. This idea of fixation has to be analysed. (For a similar view, see Glover 1970, p. 100. According to Glover, a person is unable to do otherwise if his intentions are unalterable.)

8.3 The idea of fixation

One thing is salient. Fixation does not mean the same as causal determination, although some causal sequences of events may be involved. Fixation can, in certain cases, be the result of a decision on the part of the agent. It can also, however, be the result of events over which the agent has no influence. Let me illustrate by the following example:

John is standing just below the top of Mount Etna when the volcano suddenly becomes active. John observes a stream of lava flowing quickly towards him. He realizes that if he intends to survive in this situation he must immediately run down the only existing path to the nearest village. Here a series of natural events is operating. First, the lava is flowing inexorably down the slope of the mountain. Also some mental events occur. John becomes aware of the stream of lava and he comes to the conclusion that running down the path is the only way of avoiding the stream. His intention to survive exists as a background standing condition.

I will start with the intention. The intention in this case, namely an intention to survive, is a commonplace one. But although it is almost universally present in humans it is not strictly universal. Not all people do at all moments intend to survive. Given the case that John happened to contemplate suicide at the time of the flow of the stream, running down the path would not be something he would be compelled to do.

In my example, however, John has the intention to survive. Furthermore, he has no intention to abandon it. His intention is not negotiable in favour of any other intention. Thus, John has, I would say, at least for the time being, fixated his intention to survive.

This situation could be contrasted with the following case. Peter intends to travel to Afghanistan for his holiday. He knows how to get there from his home town, he has the means for making this journey, and a perfect *PSI* with regard to it exists. Suddenly, the disaster in New York happens. The situation in the world, and in particular in Afghanistan, has changed drastically. Travelling to this country would be an insane endeavour under the circumstances. Thus Peter changes his mind. He abandons the intention to travel to Afghanistan. This means that this particular intention was a negotiable one. Thus the planned action issuing from this intention was not compelled.

But what about the other elements of the *PSI* in the case of John on Etna? Are these elements fixated – and if so, in what sense? The lava flows down and threatens John. This seems to be pure natural causation. The situational element C in the syllogism is the result of causal determination. Observe, though, that the situation C is not identical with John's becoming aware of C. For John's action to come about John must judge the lava stream to be immediately dangerous to his life.

This observation brings us to the important distinction between a sense of *objective* compulsion and a sense of *subjective* compulsion. John may misunderstand the situation and not see the danger in the stream. Then, he is not subjectively compelled. We, as observers, may, however, conclude that John is 'objectively' compelled to run down in this situation, given his basic intention to survive. Note that this sense of objective compulsion still presupposes one subjective element, namely the agent's intention. This may warrant the term 'semi-objective' to denote this variant of compulsion. We can conceive of an even more detached notion of compulsion, called the objective, ignoring also the subject's intention. A person may say, 'You are compelled to run away', not asking about John's intentions but assuming that every sensible person wants to evade any danger to his or her life.

What about the relation between C and John's becoming aware of it? Is this relation simply causal? A causal relation exists between the event in the world and the subject's perception. This is not, however, the whole story. The subject must also perform an act of interpretation. John is convinced that the lava flows down towards him. We know of cases where an agent refuses to see a fact or refuses to interpret it in the only 'objectively' reasonable way. John must accept an observation as a fact in order to act in accordance with it.

Is John's conviction that he is in mortal danger fixated in the sense we are exploring here? This question requires a complex answer since a multitude of scenarios exist. Assume that the flow of lava for some reason suddenly changes its path. The causes may be different. A rock or some trees may stand in its way, or some rescue-workers may have been quick to place obstacles in its way. As a result John observes a new fact, and he interprets it as indicating that no danger to his life exists any longer. As a result, he does not flee from the lava stream. He is no longer compelled to run. Another, but far-fetched, possibility is that John suddenly abandons his confidence in his own senses. He refuses to believe that he can be in such danger. He reinterprets his first perceptions and as a result abandons his intention to run away from the lava.

These two types of cases show that John's beliefs are not fixated. In the first type of case, he is open to revising his beliefs in the light of new perceptions. In the second type of case, he is prepared, extraordinarily, to modify his beliefs in spite of observations supporting these beliefs.

However, it could be the case that John's beliefs are fixated. The external causal story may be quite clear. No preventive factors exist. Moreover, John may be quite convinced of this story and he may not be in such a state of mind that he is even prepared to check whether rescue is on its way. He has once and for all fixated the belief that he is now in mortal danger.

What about the third factor in the syllogism: the subject's belief in necessary means for reaching the intended end? Here we can reason in a way analogous to the above. By observing and considering his situation John arrives at the conviction that the only way to avoid the stream is to run down the path on the slope as quickly as he can. Again he is observing, reasoning, and arriving at a conviction. This conviction may or may not be fixated. John may be either more or less prepared to make further observations and engage in further and alternative reasoning. If he is so prepared, his conviction is not fixated. If he is not, it is fixated.

From this we see that a person's mental abilities and attitudes are crucial for a situation of compulsion. If people have little knowledge about an area they see few alternative actions; if they have little initiative and little imagination they will never seek the alternative actions. Ignorance of alternative courses of action in order to reach an intended end thus leads to compulsion. Hence people who have less ability to see alternatives are to a greater extent than others compelled to perform the things they do.

Observe also that in many cases of decision little time is available. An action may have to be performed quickly if it is to be performed at all. Little time for negotiation is possible. No research can be undertaken. Moreover, the agent's thinking may be blocked, perhaps because of great fear or anguish. At least subjectively, no opportunity exists for renegotiating intentions or changing beliefs. Thus, in practice, because of the limitation of time, compulsion may be a reality in a number of ordinary-life situations.

With both the epistemic factors we can differentiate between objective and subjective compulsion. If we change the third component in the practical syllogism we can get an instance of 'semi-objective' compulsion in the following case: It is as a matter of fact necessary for John to run down the slope to avoid the stream and thereby save his life. Given the fixated intention of John's to save his life, he is thus semi-objectively compelled to run. My emphasis in this investigation, however, is on the subjective case. Subjective compulsion is what matters in action determination. A person acts in a certain way because he is subjectively compelled to do so, not because he is objectively or 'semi-objectively' compelled to do so.

What about the fourth factor in the syllogism? Does it have anything to do with compulsion? Is the fixation of the person's ability or opportunity relevant to this question? My answer is no. A person's ability and opportunity may change. John may break his leg on the slope and be unable to run. An obstacle may arise which prevents him from running. This, however, need not affect the situation of compulsion, either subjective or objective. Given that John finds it necessary to run down the slope to save his life, he is still compelled to run. It is a completely different matter that he will not succeed in his endeavour to run when he has broken his leg. This observation has an interesting bearing on the classical discussion on compulsion. A person may be compelled to act in a certain way, but still be unable to perform the action in question. This shows in a nutshell how different the notion of compulsion is from the notion of causal determination.

Let me summarize: Compulsion may be due to the fixation of intentions and beliefs or convictions. Subjective compulsion depends on the fixation of the agent's intentions and beliefs or convictions. Semi-objective compulsion depends on the fixation of at least one of these elements. Fixation is dependent either on natural causation or on the subject's decisions.

8.4 **The case of coercion**

What about the special case of compulsion that we call coercion, i.e. where a human being compels another human being to perform a certain action? Consider the classical case of gunpoint: a robber threatens a woman cashier and compels her to hand over the cash-box. The basic analysis is, I would say, similar. The cashier has a non-negotiable intention to survive and she has a belief that the robber might indeed kill her if she does not do what he tells her to do.

But are the beliefs and convictions non-negotiable in this case? In a way similar to the lava case they may or may not be. The cashier may reinterpret the case. She may observe that the 'robber' is a nervous young man and hardly dangerous at all. Or, she may – and this differentiates the case of human coercion from natural compulsion – start a negotiation with the man threatening her and try to persuade him to stop his foolishness. On the other hand, she may retain her initial interpretation that the situation is dangerous enough for her to succumb to the threat. In this case the initial belief remains and becomes fixated.

My description of the coercion case can be used as an introduction to the idea of various degrees of compulsion. My idea is that compulsion is not an all-or-nothing affair. One can be compelled to various degrees. I will explain.

8.5 **Compulsion as a matter of degree**

Consider, first, the case where a subject is not certain whether a threat is 'real' or not. This can also hold in the situation where the laval stream flows down the slope. John may be uncertain whether he really has to run down to save his life. He may not be able to judge the whole situation. It may well be that no real threat exists. Then, he is not subjectively compelled to run. Nevertheless, he may be overcautious and not be prepared to take any risks. He is completely convinced that his life is threatened. Thus he decides not to take any risks. In a sense he fixates a new intention, namely the one to avoid all perceived risks to his life. From this follows that he is subjectively compelled to run down the slope.

This need not be the situation, though. John need not decide not to take any risk whatsoever. Yet he may find it wise to start running. He decides to run without being strictly (subjectively) compelled to run. He may describe the situation thus: 'My choice of actions is limited to some degree. I could not walk much further up without obviously endangering my life. So I am compelled to some degree in my choice to run down the slope'.

Likewise the cashier may find her range of actions drastically narrowed in the situation of a boy threatening her with a gun. She can hardly just carry on talking to her fellow-workers or try to handle other banking matters in this situation without really raising the risk of danger both to herself and others in the bank. She is not, however, strictly compelled to hand over the money. She is only compelled to some degree.

The notion of compulsion to some degree is, however, difficult to articulate. We may claim that we are always as humans limited in our choice of actions. At this particular moment, I cannot do everything that I might like to do. I am sitting in my university building and have limited opportunities to act, at least immediately. Moreover, I have left my car at a workshop and my mobility is therefore limited. Does it, as a result of this, make sense to say that my subsequent actions are compelled to some degree?

No, it is not the limited range of actions as such that compels me. As we have seen, the notion of compulsion is tied to the concept of intention. The range of actions must be related to a particular intention. If I intend to have a meal in the university's refectory, my range of actions is not restricted. If, on the other hand, I intend to take the evening train to Stockholm my range of actions is restricted. I may, for instance, be compelled to take the next bus to the station.

However, I wish to pursue my sceptical argument further. Even if we limit ourselves to the context of a particular intention, the limitation of a range of actions is not in itself sufficient for the existence of a degree of compulsion. This suggests that the notion of compulsion (or at least the notion of a degree of compulsion) is also relative to some starting-point or some *standard*. Assume that my standard situation allows three alternative ways (*A*, *B*, and *C*) of having my lunch (which I intend to have). Assume also that this range diminishes because one of the canteens (*C*) closes down. As a result I have become compelled to choose either *A* or *B*. My subsequent choice has thereby become compelled to a higher degree, according to my suggestion.

But does not a notion of non-relative compulsion exist – that is, a notion not tied to a particular intention? Assume that I am imprisoned. I cannot move outside my cell. The satisfaction of any desire I have that concerns life outside the prison is closed to me. It seems I am compelled to remain within the cell. Do we not here encounter some non-relative sense of compulsion?

I am prevented from doing whatever I would like to do. Do we, then, need a notion of compulsion without any connection to an intention?

I think the answer is no. In the prison, I am limited with respect to a great variety of intentions. My general scope for action is extremely reduced. However, it is not completely reduced. I may have intentions concerning exercise and contemplation that I may well realize in the prison cell. However, the prison case fails to serve the purpose of illustrating a notion of absolute compulsion for a more interesting reason. Given our theory, it is not proper to say that I am compelled to remain in the cell. Remaining in the cell cannot be an intentional action if I am physically prevented from leaving the cell and I am aware of this fact.

Does this observation call for a further concept? Would it not be natural to say that a person is compelled to remain in the cell in the prison case? I think we should stick to the notion of physical force to characterize this case. Persons can be dragged from one place to another and persons can be physically bound to a certain place. In neither case do these persons perform any action. In neither case are they compelled to act in a certain way. But in both cases physical force is exerted upon them, and as a result they are prevented from acting as they desire.

So far I have talked about degrees of compulsion in terms of the limited range of actions. Further interpretations exist. I have in mind various degrees of conviction that something is a fact, either concerning the external situation or concerning means to ends. A subject may be less than convinced about a fact. In the limiting case, he or she may only suspect that something is the case. In an epistemic sense, then, the person may be described as less compelled to act in a certain direction than if he or she were convinced of the fact in question.

Earlier I distinguished between objective compulsion and subjective compulsion. I will now also make a distinction between *being subjectively compelled* and *feeling compelled*. Observe that one can be subjectively compelled in the sense of having an intention and a set of convictions with regard to necessary circumstances in order to reach an intended end *without being conscious of this fact*. My theory is compatible with the plausible assumption of unconscious wants and intentions as well as of unconscious beliefs and convictions. A person who is conscious of being subjectively compelled also *feels* the compulsion. This notion of feeling compelled is, I believe, central to certain mental illnesses.

8.6 The idea of strong desires

Now I will also test another interpretation of the notion of degrees of compulsion. This is the idea of desires of various *strengths*. In ordinary speech, we often say that John had a strong desire to do this or that he wanted very much to do that. (Observe that I do not here propose a difference between the notions of want and desire. The reason that I use the term 'desire' here is purely stylistic. In the context of urges and drives, the word 'desire' is more commonly used.) This gives a picture of a desire having a greater causal strength than other desires. How could this idea be analysed?

Consider some examples. I will first consider the 'basic' biological drives: hunger, thirst, and the sex drive. After a long period of deprivation we say that these drives must issue in a strong will to satisfy the drive in question. What is the mechanism operating here? Is it a matter of simple causal determination, of 'compulsion' in a causal necessity sense? I will argue that this is not the case although certain elements in the chain of determination are saliently causal. In the end, the person driven by his or her drive performs an intentional action. A practical syllogism is formed, containing not only the person's intention to satisfy the drive, but also the person's convictions about the best means for doing so in the situation at hand.

But what sense can be given to the 'strength' of desires? All wants, even 'weak' ones can issue in intentions. What is the difference between the strong and the weak ones? We can consider some different senses. (1) A strong desire (in the drive sense) catches the attention of the subject in many ways. Some salient and unpleasant sensations appear gradually. When we are hungry, our stomachs make themselves felt; we lose our energy; we also often get a headache. These sensations are well recognized by all human beings, who are also aware of the relief that can be achieved through having something to eat. In the case where we say that the hunger strongly compels us to get some food, the sensations are perceived by the subject to be less and less tolerable. (2) A desire may be considered strong simply in the sense that it is given first priority in the agent's mind. This may be so for the reason cited in (1), but the reason may also be purely intellectual. The agent has put this desire at the top of his or her priority list as a result of a calculation.

The two interpretations of strength of a desire have connections. A strong desire in the sensation sense tends to become a preferred desire. Hunger is normally a stronger desire for a man A than his desire to take a walk, also in the sense that if he has to choose between satisfying his hunger and his desire to take a walk, he will choose the former.

The preference analysis of strength of desires and wants has analytical and practical advantages. We can then easily order the desires in the following way: a want W is stronger for A than a want W1 if, and only if, W has a higher position on A's preference scale than W1. This holds for the basic drives, and it also holds for some other wants that we give the label 'strong'. This means that I am here proposing an analysis for the relation 'stronger than' and not for any absolute sense of strength of wants.

A third sense of a strong desire was suggested above in my discussion of people's wants and intentions to survive. Here 'strong' may mean non-negotiable or, slightly weaker, negotiable only under quite special circumstances. Under this interpretation, it is easier to give a sense to strength in the absolute sense. The completely fixated want, intention, or belief is strong. This strength then has to do with whether the intention is, and to what degree it is, fixated.

In general, all my analyses of strong desires can be subsumed under the notion of compulsion to the degree that we can talk about intentions and convictions being either more or less fixated and that there is a limited range of alternative actions to fulfil the intentions. For instance, the want that is preferred to another want is fixated to a greater degree than the want that is not.

In the light of this analysis of desires, we can understand how compulsion (or its special case coercion) need not be connected to threats or negative interactions in general. As we have seen, in particular in the discussion of Wertheimer's theory above, it has been disputed whether an *offer* can entail coercion. Can a person be said to coerce another person by offering him or her a gift or a service? An interesting and illuminating case is seduction. Can we say that a woman who sexually seduces a man coerces the man into taking part in a sexual act? In the light of my analysis, the answer is obviously yes. The woman arouses a strong desire in the man. *Ex hypothesi*, the desire is so strong that the man is not prepared to negotiate it. Hence, the desire is fixated. The man is compelled to fulfil his desire. (Consider Schramme 2004 for an interesting discussion of negative and positive cases of coercion. Schramme also comes to the conclusion that seduction can be coercive.)

8.7 On the notion of a compelling fact

So far I have only analysed the locution: *A* is compelled to do *F* in the light of *A*'s fixated intentions and convictions. An interesting further topic of investigation is locutions of the form: Situation *S* or fact *T* compelled *A* to perform *F*. The first question to ask is what factors can count as compelling.

As I have said, two elements of a *PSI*, if fixated, namely the intention and the convictions, but not the ability (see above), can function as compelling factors in the light of the rest of the *PSI*. For instance, John's intention to survive compelled him to run down the path. John's belief that the lava stream would bury him if he remained on the slope compelled him equally to run down. In this case, the two factors presuppose each other. One element is compelling in the light of the other.

We frequently also say that the external situation itself (i.e. the situation perceived in component 2 of the *PSI*) compels a person to act. In particular in a first person context, this becomes the only natural mode. I would most naturally say: the approaching car compelled me to jump away from the road. It is less natural to say: my observation of the approaching car compelled me to jump away from the road.

Can we talk, then, about compelling factors lying outside the syllogism as such? I have in mind such factors as are conditions for the elements of the *PSI*, as well as factors lying behind the fixation of our intentions and convictions. Can one, for instance, say that John's illness compelled him to act in a certain way when certain ingredients of his illness confined his thinking so that he did not see any alternative actions? Here I do not wish to legislate about language. As long as we see the difference between the primary logical relations between the elements of the *PSI* and relations between elements outside and inside the *PSI*, we maintain the theoretical clarity. Perhaps, however, the following locution is preferable: John's mental illness *caused a situation of compulsion*, since John could no longer see an alternative to the destructive course of action that he chose.

8.8 On unavoidability and ability

The perceptive reader will have observed that I have used the imperfect tense in expressing the basic formula for compulsion.

A was compelled to do *F* if, and only if, *A* could not avoid doing *F*.

My intention here is not to say that compulsion can only be detected in retrospect. I merely wish to distinguish the case of compulsion from the case of basic ability that was my topic of analysis in Part 1 of this book. The differences and similarities between the senses have come up during my discussion but in this section I will now briefly summarize my conclusions.

First, when I say that *A* could not avoid doing *F* I do not (in the general case) imply that *A* did not have the ability to avoid doing *F*. An ability statement refers to *A*'s physical and mental resources in relation to a set of standard or reasonable circumstances.

The compulsion case is very specific and is, as I have emphasized in the analysis, related to an intention and a set of beliefs. Given that *A* intends to attain *P*, and believes that doing *F* is necessary for attaining *P*, given that the intention and the belief are fixated in *A*, and given that *A* can do *F*, then *A* cannot avoid doing *F*. From my definition of the concept of intention, and on the supposition that the intention and belief are fixated all the time on the planned performance of *F*, and given that *A* can do *F*, it follows that *A* does *F*.

In the ordinary case, however, when the agent has control over the fixation of his or her intentions and can revise his or her beliefs, there is no absolute unavoidability. The unavoidability in my example is only conditional. As soon as the agent changes his or her mind, for instance makes a different decision or revises a belief that does not point in the direction of the action F, then some other action will be performed. Thus, in this standard case the agent is perfectly *capable* of avoiding doing F. It is another story that the agent may *not be prepared* to avoid doing F (which is the reason why we talk of compulsion here).

In the non-standard case when the agent does not have any control over the fixation of his or her intentions and beliefs, the situation is different. Then the agent is not able to change his or her mind in the basic sense of ability. In such a case, the agent is not capable (in the absolute sense) of avoiding doing F. This is, as I will argue in the following chapter, typical of certain mental illnesses and disorders. The inability to avoid doing a particular action F or perhaps a series of actions, for instance endless repetitive acts as in the case of obsession, may prevent the agent from realizing vital goals, such as doing systematic work or establishing deep relationships with other people. Hence my basic criteria for illness are fulfilled.

8.9 **Summary**

Now I will attempt to summarize and systematize my observations concerning compulsion.

The basic sense of compulsion which I have analysed is this:

A was compelled to do *F* if, and only if, *A* could not avoid doing *F*.

My general proposal for an analysis is the following. In the standard case, compulsion is tied to the three notions of intention, fixation, and necessity. First, a subject's action *F* is compelled in the light of an intention held by the subject; second, *F* is compelled in the light of the fact that the subject's intention and his or her convictions about circumstances and means to ends are fixated; and third, *F* is compelled in the light of the fact that *F* is considered by the subject to be a necessary means for reaching the intended end. Or to put it more formally:

A is completely subjectively compelled to do F if, and only if, *A* intends to bring about *P*, and *A* is convinced that (1) *A* is in *C* and that (2) it is necessary to perform *F* in order to bring about *P* in *C*, and *A*'s intention to bring about *P*, as well as *A*'s convictions (1) and (2), are fixated in *A*.

Fixation can come about in two ways. Agents can decide to fixate their intentions and convictions. This means that the subject may contribute to the compelling nature of the action in question. The intentions and convictions can also become fixated as a result of forces over which the agents have no control. Some mental illnesses entail delusions that often consist of beliefs that are 'forced upon the person'.

A is semi-objectively compelled to do F if, and only if, *A* intends to bring about *P*, *A* is in *C* and it is, as a matter of fact, necessary for *A* to perform *F* in order to bring about *P* in *C*.

A is subjectively compelled to some degree but less than completely subjectively compelled to *do F*, if *A* intends to bring about *P*, and *A* believes but is less than convinced that (1) and (2), and/or if *A*'s intention and convictions (1) and (2) are not completely fixated in *A*, and/or if *A* intends to bring about *P*, and *A* is convinced or believes that the range of alternative means for bringing about *P* includes more than *F* but still fewer alternatives than under standard circumstances.

A is physically forced to F if, and only if, *F* is not an action of *A*'s and *A* is prevented from abstaining from *F*.

Observe that this is a summary of the analysis of what I will call the standard type of compulsion. In the context of psychopathology, Chapter 9, I will also note a slightly different category. This category of compulsion – involving persons with severe reductions of imagination, will, or intelligence, or who suffer from a clouded consciousness – fulfils, however, the condition put down in my initial characterization: *A* was compelled to do *F* if, and only if, *A* could not avoid doing *F*.

Also observe that my analysis of compulsion is theoretical and general. It is not bound to any ethical context. In many legal and ethical contexts, compulsion is tied to the notion of *excuse*. It is a challenge to investigate what senses of compulsion (in my understanding of the word) are relevant to ethics and legislation. Here I will only make a few remarks.

We can first observe the evident fact that physical force is almost universally an excuse. If *F* is no action at all but simply a state of affairs into which the subject has been forced, then the subject cannot in general be responsible for *F*. To this there may be one notable exception. Assume that *A* has voluntarily and consciously put himself in a situation which is such (and this is known to *A*) that it involves great danger of his being subjected to physical force, either a natural physical force or force executed by robbers or other criminals. Here, there may be no excuse for performing the initial action.

What about compulsion in the action-theoretic sense? Here, as far as I can see, the excuse is to a great degree tied to *the legitimacy of the intention*. If people are compelled to perform unethical or criminal acts at gunpoint, then their acts are normally excused. Here the intention at work is the subject's intention to survive or avoid being seriously hurt. Similar intentions that may have an exculpable force are the intentions to save one's family's life and health and to save essential parts of one's property.

Another crucial question with regard to exculpation is *who* or *what* has created the fixation of the intention or beliefs in the *PSI*, or who or what has restricted the alternatives of action. If the subject has not voluntarily fixated his or her intentions or beliefs or influenced the lack of perceived alternative actions, this must be of importance for the moral and legal judgment. Reznek (1997, pp. 113–114) says: 'Automatism excuses for the same reason that ignorance and compulsion excuse – someone does not deserve moral condemnation for behaviour over which he lacks control, and for behaviour he does not know is wrong'. (For an interesting analysis of automatism not involving ideas of compulsion, see Mackie 1977.)

In the subsequent chapters, I will look further into the ways in which a subject's mental states can be involuntarily fixated.

Chapter 9

Compulsion and specific mental disorders

9.1 A meeting point for action theory and psychiatry: the phenomenon of delusion

As will have become apparent, the purpose of this book is not to contribute to psychiatry in the sense of providing causal explanations of any mental illnesses. Thus, my study differs profoundly in its purpose from, for instance, Bolton and Hill's (2003) admirable analysis of intentional and non-intentional causation of mental illness. Nor does it deal with the sharpening or, general, improvement of the diagnostic tools in psychiatry or the treatment or amelioration of mental illness. Instead, my primary concern is to discuss and clarify the relation between certain mental illnesses and agency, primarily on the part of the bearer of illness. For this purpose, I have introduced a conceptual toolkit that was first designed for ordinary action analysis. I will now attempt to show how concepts from this kit can be used for the clarification of relations between the bearer's mental illness and his or her actions.

However, I must enter traditional psychiatry from the following angles. I will use proper psychiatric examples in order to demonstrate the relevance of my toolkit. I will also use traditional psychiatric nomenclature and definitions of some crucial diagnoses. Moreover, and this is the reason for this section, I will identify and discuss the nature of some symptoms or clusters of symptoms that lie at the core of mental illness, in particular psychosis. This cluster of symptoms is usually referred to as delusions. The reason why delusions are important to me is that they are phenomena that steer the actions of mental patients in unusual and often inexplicable ways. It should be noted, however, that delusions are not the only mental states that are relevant in the following discussion.

9.1.1 Delusions – what are they?

Delusion is a key concept in psychiatry. Delusions represent what is typical for madness or insanity. Karl Jaspers (1963, p. 93) says that 'to be mad was to be deluded and indeed what constitutes a delusion is one of the basic problems of psychopathology'. Delusions signify that the subject has left rational thinking behind; he or she lacks insight; the person is in a changed state. But, more specifically, what is a delusion? The *DSM IV* defines a delusion in the following way:

> A false belief based upon incorrect inference about external reality that is firmly sustained despite what almost everyone else believes and despite what constitutes incontrovertible and obvious proof or evidence to the contrary. The belief is not one ordinarily accepted by other members of the person's culture or subculture (e.g. it is not an article of religious faith). (*DSM IV* 1994, p. 765.)

A shorter definition, but essentially in the same direction, is proposed by Buchanan and Wessely (2004, p. 242), when they say:

> The definition of delusion will follow the criteria suggested by Kräupl-Taylor (1983) and Mullen (1979) – namely that they are false beliefs, held with conviction and regarded by the subject as self-evident, which are not amenable to reason and inherently unlikely in content.

Kihlstrom and Hoyt (1988, p. 77) express themselves thus:

> Pathological delusions are anomalies of judgment or belief commonly revolving around themes of persecution, grandeur, love and jealousy, and inferiority. They are false and even implausible beliefs that are assumed to be self-evident, and they are held with intense conviction by the believer, who shows a great deal of ego-involvement and preoccupation with them. Although incorrect, and even implausible, delusions are incorrigible in the face of persuasion, counterargument, and counterdemonstration.

The latter description is the most informative and gives more details than a minimal definition. Essential ingredients in delusional beliefs are thus:

1. Falsity and implausibility
2. Held with conviction, even being incorrigible
3. A great deal of affect and ego-involvement.

There is obviously a lot of agreement in the general characterization of delusions. They are 'real' phenomena, although it is difficult to come up with the ultimate definition. However, it seems that there are problems attached to the criterion of falsity. There seem to be diagnosed delusions that are in accordance with reality. And, on the other hand, there are firmly held beliefs contrary to ordinary understanding, that are rarely taken to be signs of delusions. First, there are delusions that are obviously true even at the time of diagnosis (Fulford 1989, pp. 204–205). But, conversely, many beliefs have been judged false by the community but have afterwards been seen to be true. There is the known case of Martha Mitchell, wife of the then Attorney-General of the United States, who alleged that illegal activity involving her husband was taking place at the White House. She was considered to suffer from some psychopathology until the revelations of the Watergate affair cast new light (Maher 1988b, p. 110).

Consider also all revolutionary scientific novelties (the revolutionary medical ideas of Dr. Semmelweiss, for instance) that are normally held to be untrue by society for some time. We hardly wish to diagnose the beliefs held by such creative scientists as delusions. Moreover, falsity is a notoriously difficult notion to have as a criterion, since it can hardly ever be ultimately demonstrated. The criterion suggested by the *Oxford Textbook of Psychiatry* (Gelder et al 1989, p. 13) that delusions are unfounded beliefs is more promising.

> A delusion is a belief that is firmly held on inadequate grounds, is not affected by rational argument or evidence to the contrary, and is not a conventional belief such that the person might be expected to hold given his educational and cultural background.

The common idea that delusions are held with conviction and are almost incorrigible has also been contested. Oltmanns (1988) notes that the degree of conviction tends to fluctuate. It would, says Oltmanns, be odd to say that one and the same belief, assessed with regard to content, changes its status from being a delusion to not being so, depending on the present degree of conviction on the part of the holder.

On the other hand, most theorists tend to agree that the firm conviction is a typical property of delusions, and even Oltmanns seems to concede that all delusions (at the peak of their existence) are associated with firm conviction. Most psychiatrists also affirm the strong affect associated with a delusion. A delusion seems almost always to be of greatest importance to the sufferer.

This brings us to noting what Kihlstrom and Hoyt (1988) contend, namely that delusions are hardly any old beliefs. Their content typically concerns the subject to a high degree. They centre around the ego. They typically revolve around persecution, grandeur, love, jealousy, and inferiority. Spitzer (1988) expresses the aspect of subject-centredness in a different way. He describes delusions as statements formally on a par with 'I am in pain' and other utterances that express subjective mental states. However, their explicit content may concern accessible (objective) facts.

All these general themes tend to be universal. On the other hand, the specific contents of the beliefs can be culture-relative. Westermeyer (1988, p. 218) sums up the literature by saying: 'The structure of delusions varies little, if any, across cultures, whereas the content may be influenced by culture. In developing countries, culture-bound aspects of delusional content involve principally religious and traditional culture-bound world views, especially those that are being undermined by modern secular society'.

Must delusions be beliefs that can be true or false? This common assumption is challenged by Fulford (1989; 2004), who claims that value judgements can also be delusions. One may then wonder how they can be judged. The idea must be that the value judgement is totally unsupported, for instance, when a father says that his daughter is highly immoral without having any basis for that judgment. Value judgements are like beliefs in the sense that they call for factual support.

In the summing up of criteria of delusions, Oltmanns (1988, p. 5) mentions the following characteristics, none being considered as either necessary or sufficient:

a. The balance of evidence for and against the belief is such that other people consider it completely incredible.

b. The belief is not shared by others.

c. The belief is held with firm conviction. The person's statements or behaviours are unresponsive to the presentation of evidence contrary to the belief.

d. The person is preoccupied with (emotionally committed to) the belief and finds it difficult to avoid thinking or talking about it.

e. The belief involves personal reference, rather than unconventional religious, scientific, or political conviction.

f. The belief is a source of subjective distress or interferes with the person's occupational or social functioning.

g. The person does not report subjective effort to resist the belief (in contrast to patients with obsessional ideas).

Criterion c is crucial for our reasoning. The person's beliefs seem to be fixated and unable to be altered by the person him- or herself even in the face of overwhelming contrary evidence. Moreover, criterion f says that the belief is a source of subjective distress or interferes with the person's functioning. Here, we find our essential condition for the delusion's constituting a state of illness.

9.1.2 Where are delusions to be found? And where do they come from?

As I have noted above, delusions have been considered the central symptoms of insanity and are crucial criteria of psychosis today. In *DSM IV*, they are grouped under such headings as: Bizarre, Persecutory, Grandiose, Poverty, Jealousy, Reference, Nihilistic, and Somatic. Current measurements such as The Present State Examination (PSE) acknowledge 13 different kinds of delusion and The Schedule for Affective Disorders and Schizophrenia (SADS) gives 11 types. The most common ground for division among delusions is the content of the delusion. Some attempts have been made, however, to distinguish between delusions from the point of view of their logical structure. A classical proposal was made by Southard (1916). For a discussion, see Maher (1988a).

Delusions occur in many mental conditions. *Ex hypothesi*, they can be found in all psychoses, primarily in schizophrenia, where delusion is a direct marker.

They are also common in bipolar diseases. Delusions of grandiosity are typical for the state of mania, whereas delusions of guilt, inferiority, and poverty are typical of the state of depression. However, delusions have been reported as ingredients in as many as 70 conditions, including several somatic ones (Maher 1988a). They range all the way from neurological syndromes to metabolic and endocrine disorders to syndromes associated with alcohol and other drugs.

What are the theories about the origin and aetiology of delusions? The theories vary considerably.

a. Cognitive accounts. A plausible idea is that there is a defect in the reasoning faculty of the subject. The delusion is taken to be a result of faulty reasoning. There is little evidence, however, that persons with delusions are impaired concerning the ability of basic logical reasoning. Some tests have been performed in this regard by Chapman and Chapman. These authors find on the other hand that some subjects tend to 'jump to conclusions' on the basis of quite weak premises. They also seem to constrict the information used in reaching a conclusion. They appear to have a tendency to cling to a belief that they really wish to hold (in mania) or greatly fear (in depression, schizophrenia, and paranoia).

b. Motivational accounts. These accounts date from the early Freudian theories. Psychoanalysts have suggested that delusions are projections of personal inner, unconscious states (for instance, unfulfilled wishes or unresolved conflicts) onto external sources. A contemporary theorist, Neale (1988), has used psychoanalytic ideas in providing an aetiological account of grandiose delusions in mania. He claims that unstable self-esteem is a predisposition to such delusions.

c. Perceptual theories. Maher (1974 and 1988a and b) is a strong proponent of the idea that delusions mainly stem from abnormal perceptions. Maher thereby distances himself mainly from the cognitive/reasoning account. In a 1974 article, he says that delusional thinking is not itself aberrant. This means that delusions are basically formed in the same way as ordinary beliefs. Moreover, delusions ought to be looked upon as theories. They are theories that are called for in order to explain odd perceptual data. The fact that they explain the data well is a reason why the subject so strongly clings to them. In this, the delusioned people do not distingush themselves from ordinary scientists, who indeed often cling to their favourite theories even in the face of contradictory data.

9.1.3 New ideas about the nature and source of delusions

In two recent studies (Stephens and Graham 2004, and Gipps and Fulford 2004), some basic assumptions in the traditional research on delusions have been challenged. Stephens and Graham contest the idea that delusions need be beliefs at all. They cite certain accounts saying that people with delusions often do not exhibit the emotive responses that beliefs would lead us to expect. A patient may have reported that his wife is trying to kill him while remaining completely indifferent. Others report that delusions often fail to engage behaviour. Although the patient claims that a terrible fact is true, he or she sometimes does not at all act on the claim. As a consequence, Stephens and Graham think we need a different theory of delusions taking account of the fact that some delusions appear to be firmly held beliefs whereas others are not. Their solution entails introducing a hierarchy of mental states. What is common to persons with delusions, they say, is a delusional stance, i.e. an attitude towards a lower-order epistemic state (not necessarily of the belief kind) sketched in the following way:

> S is deluded that p, just in case p is the representational content of a lower-order state or attitude of S: (a) with which S personally identifies, (b) to which S clings in the face of strong contrary considerations, and (c) about which S lacks insight into the nature and imprudent costs of maintaining. (p. 240)

Gipps and Fulford (2004) also challenge the traditional way of viewing delusions. Delusions are not necessarily beliefs that are the results of an act of reasoning starting at the stage of perception. Gipps and Fulford, influenced by phenomenologists such as Merleau-Ponty, propose a different conception of the mind, called an *engaged* epistemology, which entails that there is not (or need not be) a reasoning from perception to belief. Instead, the typical experience of the world already contains in itself an understanding of the world. Our way of understanding, they claim, is not mediated by some kind of reasoning. We know the world directly in our experience. Gipps and Fulford make a point of emphasizing that delusions can have different ontological characters; apart from beliefs, they may be direct experiences, but also moods, feelings, and evaluations.

John Cutting (1999) is an author who offers an original account of delusions based on an elaborate general theory of psychopathology. I cannot do justice here to his comprehensive exposition, where he combines philosophical insights with contemporary neuropsychological hypotheses. I will just briefly present his basic view on the nature of delusions.

Two fundamental concepts in Cutting's theory of mind are reason and intuition. Reason is the mental faculty that 're-presents' the world. It is the faculty that categorizes and characterizes (conceptually and linguistically) a thing in the world. Intuition, on the other hand, is the faculty that invests a thing with value, i.e. identifies the thing as having a positive or negative value. To invest with value often entails becoming aware of something as inviting one's concern.

Typically, it is intuition that starts an inquiry: I am curious about this. What is it? As an answer comes an explanation of what it is. This explanation is given by reason, either the subject's own faculty of reason or the reason of someone else.

Cutting's neuropsychological hypothesis, corroborated by several empirical findings, is that the left hemisphere of the brain is largely responsible for rational thinking, i.e. reason, and that the right hemisphere is the site of intuition. Normally, the left and the right hemisphere of the brain interact harmoniously. This means that reason and intuition support each other. But both hemispheres and both faculties can be disturbed. This is indeed the case with delusions, Cutting contends. It is characteristic of delusions that both reason and intuition are impaired. What is presented to intuition is anomalous, and what is represented by reason is more deranged than it would have been if reason were just rationalizing the anomalous representation.

> The problem in the realm of intuition is exactly the same as ... in the case of pure anomalous experiences. The whole qualitative matrix of the world, as presented to intuition before anything is experienced, is altered, and in such a way that no quality is presented in the sort of way that it is presented to a normal person.... For the subject, the world is presented in another way. That is why the subject reacts with perplexity or terror – a delusional mood, in traditional terms – to the completely new state of affairs. Over time, reason represents this in the only way it can – in the terms of the socially available explanations at its disposal: someone has poisoned me, a world war is going on, etc. A delusion is the judgement of reason on the anomalous state of affairs thrown up by intuition. (Cutting 1999, pp. 258–259)

The authors of these three studies modify the traditional picture of delusions in crucial ways. In one basic respect, however, they remain faithful to the current idea of delusions. They agree with the traditionalists that delusions are mental states that have some cognitive content. Even if these states are not beliefs in a traditional specific sense of the word, they are some other mental states: experiences, understandings or attitudes, which directly or indirectly take some proposition as their object. This proposition need not be theoretical; it can be an evaluative or normative proposition. However, this proposition, whatever its status, can be assessed. And it is precisely this proposition that can be assessed, for instance, in the psychiatric case, as being unusual, bizarre, or even irrational. Hence, these modern views of delusions do not change the basic picture from the point of view of my present analysis.

Musalek (2003) highlights a different aspect of delusions, namely their meanings. He differentiates between the meanings of the delusional content, the meanings of suffering from a delusion as a mental disorder, and the meanings of particular behaviours of deluded patients. Musalek notes that the delusional world is always a meaningful world to its bearer. The deluded person is, as well as we all are to some extent, thrown into an ambiguous and precarious world.

A vulnerable person may respond to this world by creating a fairly unambiguous and stable, but delusional, world as an act of defence. The presentation of the delusional world to others, however, often leads to misunderstandings. Such misunderstandings can in their turn reinforce and prolong delusional convictions and thereby establish the condition as a chronic disorder. Bolton and Hill (2003, pp. 332–333) support this hermeneutic (or, as they say, intentional) interpretation of many delusions. '…the symptoms at least of some sufferers may be seen as the outcome of coping strategies which restore coherence to representations and provide a basis for action'.

In using the term 'the meaning of suffering from a delusion', Musalek refers to the deluded person's interpretation of and suffering from the prejudices of relatives, acquaintances, and colleagues. The notion of 'meaning of particular behaviours' is explained in the following way:

> For example, patients suffering from delusions of persecution are usually suspicious about the people surrounding them and suppose them to be possible persecutors. Uncertain as to whether these people are persecutors or not, patients suffering from delusions of persecution interact with them not only verbally but also para-verbally and non-verbally, in a very special way. The behaviour and communication style of the patients may lead to particular reactions in people they relate to. People who are usually very open and friendly with others may react to the deluded patient with some reservation and resentment because of the patient's suspicious behaviour. This serves to reinforce the suspicions of the patient. (p. 166)

In general, Musalek contends, it is the social interactions and the emotions created by such interactions that determine the course of the delusional disorder. If the interaction is negative, full of misunderstandings and suspicions, then the negative emotions of fear, anguish, and anger are reinforced, and so is the condition. This, in its turn, leads to a loss of freedom. 'The patient suffering from delusional ideas is no longer able to decide what he or she wants to do: the delusional convictions move the patient' (Musalek 2003, p. 157). This is particularly true of the delusions of persecution and the paranoic disorders to which I shall return below.

9.1.4 Concluding points about delusions

As will have become evident, it is difficult to find a comprehensive definition of delusions about which everybody can agree. There are, however, certain features that are common to most characterizations of delusions. For my own purposes in this book, I can summarize these features in the following way.

First, delusions are (at least partly) cognitive states of a person. We mostly refer to them as beliefs, but they can be other states (experiences, understandings, or attitudes) that have some cognitive content. Second, the content of such a cognitive state is typically considered to be unusual or even bizarre by most people.

Third, the cognitive state is normally held with strong conviction. This conviction is often maintained by the person despite strong contrary evidence. Moreover, the person typically cannot avoid having the cognitive state even if he or she would like to change it.

9.2. **General remarks on mental illness and compulsion**

It became apparent in the discussion in Chapter 7 that much of the irrationality encountered in mental illness is compelled, in some sense, something that the subject cannot help or avoid having or doing. In ordinary life, many cases exist where irrationality is deliberately chosen. A person can choose to believe something stupid and can choose to behave in a way that is irrational to most of my senses. Such choices need not be a sign of illness (except for the case where the choice in itself is compelled).

In my analysis above (Chapter 8), I noted that the notions of fixation and necessity are central to compulsion. I also noted that the range of alternatives open to the agent determines the degree of compulsion with which he or she performs an action. The range of alternative actions that are open to the subject who is compelled has become limited. In a particular situation, a set of factors limits the subject's choice of actions. In the 'perfect' case of compulsion, the subject can choose only one action: if A was compelled to perform F, then A could not perform anything else than F. In a weak sense, at least, A's performing F is determined.

My analysis of the standard case of compulsion can be summarized in the following way: The sentence 'A is compelled to do F' means that a goal P exists such that A has a *fixated* intention to achieve P, and a *fixated* conviction that F is an action that is necessary to perform in order to attain P. Two important elements exist in this analysis: (i) an intention and some convictions that are in some sense fixated, and (ii) the action F as considered by the subject to be necessary in order to achieve the intended end.

First, what is the sense of this fixation? It can be viewed both in an abstract, suppositional, way and in a concrete, physical, way. The former is the case if we express ourselves as follows. I will assume Tom's intention to go to Stockholm by train this afternoon as something given; then Tom is compelled to take the 4 o'clock train, since that is the only train to Stockholm this afternoon. The fixation here is the fixation of a thought experiment. The agent need not then be 'really' compelled to take the train. He may indeed change his mind about going to Stockholm.

The situation becomes more interesting when we consider the intention as being as a matter of fact fixated. This could be the case in two ways. One is the case where an agent has *decided* to fixate his or her intentions. He or she is then not prepared to relinquish these intentions, whatever the circumstances. This is typically the case with our most important intentions, such as the one to defend our lives, whatever the circumstances. The other main case is the one where an agent has an intention or a set of convictions or beliefs that he or she cannot avoid having. The intention or the conviction is in a way forced upon the subject, and the subject cannot get rid of it through his or her own decision-making. With regard to this intention or this conviction, the agent cannot change his or her mind.

The first general case where the subject decides to fixate the intention and is not prepared to relinquish it is probably the most common case when we talk about compulsion in ordinary affairs. The paradigm example here is the one of being forced at gunpoint. A woman cashier is not prepared to relinquish her intention to survive. In the situation of being at gunpoint, she sees no way of securing survival but by following the gunman's orders.

This case of compulsion has by itself nothing to do with mental disorder or mental illness. It is a frequent phenomenon in everybody's life. However, certain cases of mental illness exist (where the illness is identified independently of the phenomenon of compulsion) that exhibit as a typical element a state of compulsion according to this standard analysis. I will return to such a case below.

As I have said, the intentions that are fixated by will concern one's vital interests. These typically deal with one's own safety, with the safety of one's nearest and dearest, and of one's most important property. But nothing in principle limits the vital interests to this basic sector. A man can have a vital interest in the form of a non-negotiable intention of raising his income to at least $5 million a year. Because of this, he may be compelled to do many things, some of which may be morally reproachable. This notion of compulsion is thus not a notion that can automatically be used for moral or legal purposes, for instance for the purpose of exculpating the subject. It is a theoretical notion based on the simple relation to the idea of a fixated intention. Lawrie Reznek notes this case when he speaks of people who are strong-minded and idealistic. 'They cannot be deterred from their course of action, even by the threat of the law ... The fact that their intention is unalterable does not mean that they are incapable of doing otherwise and not responsible for their actions' (1997, pp. 85–86). (Observe that the person at gunpoint is also able to do otherwise, but is still not responsible.)

Many intentions and convictions talked about so far are, strictly speaking, avoidable from the subject's point of view. The subjects *can* abandon them, i.e withdraw their fixation, although they may *not want* to abandon them. The man in my example can, in principle, abandon his intention to earn $5 million; a woman can abandon her intention to save her property and can even abandon her intention to survive. Indeed, we know of people who decide to take their lives or make no effort to resist the process of dying. The same holds for many but not all convictions held by a person.

The situation is different when the intention or conviction is such that a person cannot avoid having it. These mental states are, as we say, forced upon the person, who has never decided to have them; moreover, the force remains constant throughout some period of time, so that during this period the person becomes compelled to perform all those actions that he or she considers necessary for the realization of the fixated intention in question.

Do salient examples of this case exist? The case of strong drives, either natural, such as hunger or thirst, or artificial, such as those induced by drugs, might qualify. We often express ourselves in terms of compulsion here. The persons who have starved are compelled to eat and the persons who are on drugs are compelled to satisfy their drives. This situation could be described in the following way. The subjects have an intention that is forced upon them, and they cannot get rid of it. They consider a particular action F to be necessary for realizing the intended end. Thus, these persons cannot avoid doing F.

In the theory of psychiatry, one often encounters the case where a belief is forced upon the subject, like in the case of delusions discussed in the previous section. A woman cannot avoid believing, for instance, that some dangerous animal has appeared in her garden. Even if this woman performs a rational deliberation to the effect that a dangerous animal cannot reasonably be present, she retains the irrational belief. Such a situation can induce a compelled action in the light of a standing intention on the part of the subject. If she intends to protect her life and security, she must take measures for this protection in the light of her belief. Hence, her action to call the police or to fetch a gun can be conceived of as a compelled action. This case is then analogous to the former case, but a reverse fixation occurs. In the former case, the *intention* was fixated by force. Here, the *belief* is fixated by force. This is the typical case of a delusion, i.e. a belief that can be retained and remain fixated in spite of overwhelming arguments against it.

So far, I have attempted to identify examples of compulsion where an intention or a belief is 'forced' upon an agent. In many of these examples, the agents can (at least at times) see and know that the actions that are performed by them are irrational or stupid. Thus, the agents in these cases have normally retained a basic rationality in their thinking. A paranoiac can, of course, have a completely rational hierarchy of goals, and have a very sharp and lively intellect too; the only thing is that his or her notion of reality is in one specific respect utterly distorted. Apart from the drive, the kleptomaniac or pyromaniac can be similarly rational in their thinking. What has happened is that their basic rationality is no longer controlling their actions. (For a discussion, see Fried and Agassi 1976.)

Consider now a slightly different category, one that is probably rather common in the statistics of criminality. I have in mind persons with very low intellectual agility and a poor capacity, or even no capacity at all, for weighing one goal against another. Normally, their goals are quite rudimentary and unlikely to be enriched. How should their behaviour be viewed from our present point of view?

In order to simplify the argument, consider quite an extreme case. Assume that a man has the goal of satisfying a basic drive to kill a little boy. Assume also that he does not see, and indeed does not even have the capacity to see, any goal, moral or otherwise, which is in conflict with this goal. As a matter of brute fact, his goal is not then open to negotiation. He, therefore, kills the boy in order to satisfy his drive and cannot see any alternative to this behaviour in order to achieve the satisfaction of the drive.

Does this case fulfil the condition of compulsion? The case is in many ways different from the cases previously discussed. In these, the problem was the fixation, either of an intention or of a conviction. In the present case, the problem is that there appears to be no repertoire of alternative intentions or beliefs to choose from. The person is amoral and completely unimaginative. Since no alternative goal was available he could not have acted otherwise than he did. Thus, this case satisfies the basic general criterion of compulsion. But it belongs to a second type of compulsion. Compulsion, I will now say, is either dependent on the fixation of an intention or a conviction, in the sense that an intention or a conviction has been installed and maintained by the subject or some external force, or it is dependent on *a lack of alternatives* to an intention or a conviction. The two cases have one crucial thing in common. The pair intention/conviction is completely determined in the situation of action.

Alternative actions can be blocked for further reasons. Consider the case of overwhelming anger (as in provocation) and of overwhelming fear (as in some cases of duress). (For further discussion, see Reznek 1997, p. 79.) A man who is extremely angry, for instance because he has been prevented from attaining an important goal, may be compelled from the point of view of a fixated intention. But a further element can be added to this. His overwhelming emotion blocks his thinking. He cannot consider any actions alternative to the one he sets himself to perform. We can find a parallel reasoning for the case of fear. Fear is related to the safety of one's body and what one holds dear. Here are some fixated intentions. But, in addition to this, the emotion as a psychological phenomenon, as something which blocks thinking, can play a role in the situation of compulsion.

The situation where there is no repertoire of alternative actions available to the subject can perhaps be even more clearly illustrated by certain cases of brain damage or lesions due to neurological diseases. Patients suffering from so-called *utilization behaviour syndrome* can repeatedly perform completely irrational intentional actions, not being inhibited by the obvious nonsense of the behaviour. The classic example is the man who, every time he sees a pair of glasses on a table, picks them up and puts them on. This is done even if he is already wearing a great number of pairs of glasses. Such a series of nonsense actions will, in the extreme case, never be stopped by the agent himself. (See Marchetti and della Sala 1998.)

Here, it seems as if the subject cannot help iterating the irrational behaviour. A plausible interpretation of this situation is that no alternative repertoire of actions is available, given, for instance, the fixated intention to wear a pair of glasses. The subject does not realize the existence of any alternative action (at least not in the circumstances presented). Thus, the subject is unable to do anything else than what he or she actually does.

One might, in some instances, dispute whether persons suffering from the utilization syndrome really perform intentional actions. However, the behaviour in question is clearly goal-directed and is informed by convictions or beliefs (in our example, the adequate belief that a pair of glasses lies in front of the person). Thus, these persons seem to fulfil the basic conditions of intentionality presented above.

Similar considerations can be applied to the phenomenon called *automatism*, as described in certain psychiatric contexts. Reznek (1997, p. 93) states that the following legal definition of automatism was given in a case called Bratty's appeal: '[Automatism] means unconscious, involuntary action, and it is a defence because the mind does not go with what is being done ... [One could] explain automatism simply as action without any knowledge of acting, or action with no consciousness of doing what was being done.' According to this definition, automatic 'acts' would hardly qualify as actions at all. However, the issue is controversial. Schopp (1991, pp. 135–136) gives the following characterization: 'Automatism cases sometimes involve acts done in a skilled, coordinated manner, apparently for the purpose of achieving some specific end. ... [T]hese facts seem to indicate that the actors knew what they were doing and acted as they did precisely for the purpose of performing the act constituting the objective elements of the offense.' A plausible characterization of this case could follow the analysis of the utilization syndrome. The behaviour in question is intentional, but the agent is not aware of any alternative course of action. Thus, the activity in question satisfies the conditions for being compelled.

Schopp argues in a similar manner. What is significant in cases of automatism, he says, is that these people have their consciousness impaired, not in the sense that their behaviour is unintended but in the sense that they have limited access to their own standing wants and beliefs. In ordinary deliberation, says

Schopp, we have continuous access to the whole of our stock of wants and beliefs and can at least roughly check what the consequences will be of a particular choice of action in relation to other wants and beliefs.

A person who acts in a state of impaired consciousness is acting in a state of distorted awareness and attention such that his acts may be caused by an action plan, but the plan is selected with access to only a small and nonrepresentative portion of his wants and beliefs. The actor's wants and beliefs do not cause his acts, therefore, in the manner characteristic of ordinary human activity. (p. 145)

Let me try to summarize this category of people whom we may describe as being compelled to act in a certain way, owing to the non-availability of alternative actions in a specific situation. This non-availability can be due to different factors and can be described in slightly different ways. Common to the person with utilization syndrome behaviour, the intellectually limited person and the person who exhibits automatism is, however, that they do not see that they can or should do anything else than they actually do. In the extreme case of utilization syndrome behaviour, the person literally has no access to an alternative behaviour. The person with limited intellectual agility may see the existence of alternative actions but has no ability for calculating the consequences that may in the long run damage him or her. The person with 'clouded consciousness' due to disease may similarly have lost the ability to calculate but has typically lost the ability to get access to his or her whole stock of wants and beliefs that may be relevant for decision and action in the situation at hand.

9.3 A study of some psychiatric diagnoses involving compulsion

9.3.1 The paradigm case of paranoia

The basic import of my analysis of compulsion is that a circumstance, which could be consituted by an action performed by some other agent, is compelling to an agent if there is no set of alternative actions, of the various kinds discussed above, open to the agent in the light of his or her intentions and beliefs. A paradigm case of compulsion in ordinary affairs is, as I have said, the bank robbery at gunpoint. Here, the set of alternative actions is closed because of the non-negotiablility of the agent's basic intention to survive. The robbery is a case of compulsion, since the clerk intends to survive and she is not prepared to relinquish this intention. And, given the circumstances, she sees that the only secure way to survive is to hand over the money. The question now is if this kind of case can have a bearing on the analysis of some mental illness.

An obvious parallel exists in some of the clear cases of paranoia. (I will use the term 'paranoia' here, although its suitability has been disputed (see Munro 1998).

The presently favoured diagnostic term, also in *DSM IV*, appears to be 'delusional disorder'. It should then also be emphasized that delusional disorders need not be of the persecutory type of which I am giving an example here. Other subtypes of delusional disorder are pathological jealousy and paraphrenia. Moreover, delusions of the persecutory type are also frequent in other disorders such as paranoid schizophrenia and mood disorders). Consider the paranoid man who believes that his life is threatened. Subjectively, the paranoiac is in the same situation as the bank clerk; he sees his life as being threatened, and sees perhaps only one way of parrying the threat. Thus, he is forced or compelled to perform an action that he considers to be the only possible one in order to avoid the threat to his life. The significant difference between the latter case and the one of the bank clerk is that the bank clerk's threat is real (a robber really stands beside him), whereas the threat in the case of paranoia is purely 'imagined'. No person is persecuting the paranoiac. The paranoiac is only subjectively threatened. However, from the point of view of the rationalization of the action, i.e. in terms of the *PSWs* preceding the actions, a complete parallel exists. In this sense, we can say that the paranoiac's action is an *internally compelled* action.

A classic case exists in the history of forensic psychiatry, illustrating exactly this situation of compulsion. This case has given its name to a classic rule in British criminal law, called the *M'Naghten rules*. M'Naghten had killed the secretary of Robert Peel, the British Prime Minister, in 1843. It came out at the trial that it was actually the Prime Minister himself that M'Naghten had intended to kill, the motive being provided by his deluded idea that he was persecuted by the Tories. He thought that the only way to put a stop to this persecution was to murder Peel. M'Naghten was acquitted on account of his mental aberration. (For a detailed account of this case, see Radden 1985.)

Thus, we seem to have a case of compulsion from the arena of mental illness that fulfils my technical criteria of compulsion. The question can now be put: is the compelling nature of the paranoiac's action a significant feature of the illness of paranoia or delusional disorder? Is this a sufficient criterion of paranoia? No, this does not seem to be the case. Many actions exist, performed in the ordinary course of affairs by normal adults, which are internally compelled (without the existence of an external threat). There are all the cases where we *mistakenly* believe that something very threatening occurs and thus act in the manner we consider necessary in order to avoid the threat. We may even be completely justified in our belief. Consider the following case: An officer at war has been taught how to recognize an enemy tank. He is one day in an observation position and discovers a tank coming in his direction, displaying the enemy's emblem. He thinks that he has been discovered by the enemy and, therefore, orders fire on the tank in order to protect his base. Afterwards, it is discovered that it was not really the enemy who was approaching. Some of the officer's own troops had gotten hold of an enemy tank and had forgotten to report this to him.

Here is a case of internal compulsion without an external counterpart. This, however, is neither an instance of paranoia nor of any other mental illness. A mistaken belief is not in itself a sign of illness. Nor is an unjustified mistaken belief a sufficient criterion of illness. The paranoiac is ill, not simply because he or she is compelled (or feels compelled) to kill a person because of a mistaken belief. The person is ill basically because he or she is *unable to avoid* a certain kind of mistaken belief. (The officer in my example is still able to change his belief in the face of new evidence.) The rationality in the belief formation is deranged. But it is true that the case becomes a case of a *serious* illness since the belief is of such a kind as to compel the subject to commit an appalling crime and thus something that goes against his vital goals in the long run. Fried and Agassi (1976, p. 72) write: 'The paranoic lives in a private world and speaks in a private language. He treats his own idiosyncratic integrative principle the way most people treat the publicly accepted – institutionalised – one, and is almost totally oblivious of or summarily dismisses the publicly accepted one, at least on points of conflict'.

Paranoia entails having some delusion. The analysis made so far for the case of paranoia can be generalized to the whole area of delusions. (See my characterization of delusions in Section 9.2) Allow me to, with the help of Leff and Isaacs (1990, p. 50), pursue the examination of delusions further. The authors first make a distinction between full and partial delusion. 'Patients who concede under questioning that their delusions might be mistaken, due to their imagination, or part of a psychiatric illness, are suffering from *partial delusions*. Patients whose false beliefs cannot be shaken by argument have *full delusions*. It is essential to view the patient's beliefs in relation to the information available to him and to the beliefs that are current in his cultural group'.

Some of the subspecies of delusion recognized by Leff and Isaacs (1990) are the following:

1. *Delusion of thought insertion.* 'The patient experiences thoughts in his mind which he does not recognize as originating in his own thought processes' (p. 52).

2. *Delusion of thought broadcast.* 'The patient feels that his thoughts are transmitted to other people' (p. 53).

3. *Delusion of thought withdrawal.* 'The patient experiences a sudden interruption in his train of thought. This occurs without warning and is out of the patient's control' (p. 54).

4. *Delusion of control.* 'In the group of symptoms included in delusions of control, the patient experiences some outside force or power as replacing, partly or wholly, his control over one or more of these mental activities' (p. 55).

5. *Delusional perception.* 'The symptom consists of two stages; first the patient focuses on a particular percept, and then he suddenly realizes that the percept has immense personal significance for him. The link made by the patient between the initial perception and its significance is not understandable or logical to anyone else' (p. 57).

6. *Paranoid delusion.* 'These are the commonest types of delusion and may occur in any of the functional or organic psychoses or may exist as an isolated symptom. The patient believes that a person, a group of people, or some supernatural force is intent on harming him when there is no basis for this in reality' (p. 58). (Munro (1998) would prefer to talk here about persecutory delusions.)

7. *Delusion of reference.* 'The patient sees references to himself in communications which in reality could not possibly be meant for him. ... If the patient hears remarks addressed to him only when other people are present and attributes the remarks to them, he has a delusion of reference and *not* auditory hallucinations' (p. 60).

8. *Delusion of misidentification and misinterpretation.* 'The patient holds mistaken beliefs about the identity of people or places, or misinterprets the nature of situations. ... Occasionally patients express the belief that their close relatives have been replaced by imposters who look identical' (p. 61).

9. *Grandiose delusion.* 'These occur typically in mania, but are also found in schizophrenia and the organic psychoses. There may also be a grandiose element in the delusions associated with depressive psychosis, for example, the patient's conviction that he has brought disaster to the whole world' (p. 62).

10. *Delusion of guilt.* 'Depressed patients commonly express guilt about things they believe they have done in the past ... but to be assessed as delusional it has to be out of all proportion to the patient's acts. There are usually three components to delusions of guilt: the patient exaggerates the nature of his bad deeds, he believes he has done a disproportionate amount of harm to the people he loves, and he anticipates some terrible punishment which he feels he deserves' (p. 63).

11. *Religious delusion.* 'These raise particular problems of differentiation from subcultural beliefs. Some beliefs are obviously delusional; that the patient

is God, the Virgin Mary, Christ, or a saint. But others, such as the patient's conviction that he has a special relationship with God or that God communicates with him, can be hard to distinguish from beliefs current in minority religious groups to which he may belong' (p. 65).

I present this list here without further analysis. It is not clear, however, that all the listed species fall under the general definition of delusion (see above). Consider, for instance, delusion of thought withdrawal. If one experiences an interruption of a train of thought, it appears that there must indeed be some interruption. Why should this phenomenon be labelled a delusion?

9.3.2 Some other forms of compulsive psychiatric disorder: kleptomania, pyromania, drug addiction

Certain other psychiatric conditions exist that are signified by the fact that the subject is (or feels) 'compelled' to do something. Again, this compulsion is not of the ordinary external kind, exemplified by the case of the bank clerk. The compulsion is purely internal. Something within the person 'forces' him or her to perform a certain action. Typically, such actions are shoplifting (*kleptomania*), burning down houses (*pyromania*), and the taking of drugs.

Reznek (1997, p. 83) describes the condition of kleptomania in the following way: 'kleptomaniacs lack the ability to do otherwise because when faced with the prospect of being imprisoned (a standard change in circumstances) they do not desist'.

Is it here really a case of compulsion in my technical sense? Or is it some other kind of situation for which the metaphor 'compulsion' may seem adequate? Is it possible to generalize from the case of the paranoiac, to extend this paradigm to other cases of inner compulsion, for instance to the type of compulsion that is more in the nature of a drive? Parallels are often drawn in the psychiatric literature between the compulsion encountered in neuroses, such as like kleptomania and pyromania, on the one hand, and basic physiological drives such as hunger and sexuality on the other. (cf. my points about drives above in the general analysis of compulsion, Chapter 8, Section 8.6.)

It may appear at first glance that a great difference exists between the experience of a drive and the experience of a threat, but I think a case exists for proposing basically the same analysis of these conditions. Two phenomena exist that have a central position with regard to the determination of acts by drives. In the first place, every unsatisfied drive is a cause of discomfort, often in the form of a tension. In the second place, an agent often knows from experience what the satisfaction of the drive bears with it in the form of a pleasant sensation. Most people have set intentions that, *prima facie*, motivate drive satisfaction. The most extreme type of such intention is that of maximizing pleasure.

Less extreme types concern the maintenance of a physical state of relative peace and harmony. When it comes to the basic drives of hunger, thirst, and sex, the picture also includes intentions that ultimately concern the continued existence of the subject and of the human race. Feelings of hunger and thirst, for instance, can become intolerable to the subject. He or she wants in the first place to get rid of them. However, a more basic intention, namely the one to survive, may also come into play. In both cases, the intentions are preformed, and the subject is not prepared to negotiate them.

Now, are these sensations compelling in my technical sense? They can be so if the persons who have the drives are not prepared to abandon or modify their intentions (for instance, in the light of a conflict with duty or with another basic goal). On the other hand, it is far from certain that they are compelling in the sense that morality or jurisprudence can regard them as exculpatory. For instance, a person's intention to maximize his pleasure cannot without further ado be accepted as an exculpatory one. A considerably more plausible candidate as an exculpatory intention is where the agent wants to free him- or herself of a very strong or even unbearable tension. If psychiatry does think that the sensations experienced by the kleptomaniac or pyromaniac, whose drive remains unsatisfied, are unbearably uncomfortable or unbearably importunate, then it is reasonable to look on these sensations as morally legitimizing, to look upon them as constituting imperative reasons for the act by which the drive is satisfied.

The question of illness arises again. Does the compelling nature of the actions by the kleptomaniac, the pyromaniac, or the drug addict determine their status as illnesses? I think here that the logic of illness should be explained in the following way. The subject has a drive that he or she cannot (in the short run) avoid. The drive in itself is forced upon the subject. This drive is very strong indeed, in the sense that it seems unbearable to the subject not to satisfy it. The subject is then 'compelled' to satisfy it. The satisfaction of the drive is in conflict with some of the subject's vital goals. Satisfying the drive to steal little things from the store, in the case of the kleptomaniac, prevents the subject from fulfilling his or her duty to be a law-abiding citizen. Hence, the subject is unable, in this case, to realize one of his or her vital goals. Thus, the subject is ill.

9.3.3 Obsessions

Leff and Isaacs (1990, p. 88) define obsessional acts in the following way: 'These are repetitive acts, usually commonplace in nature, which the patient feels compelled to carry out, although he resists them as unnecessary or even stupid'. Charlton (1988, p. 158) gives the following more comprehensive account: 'In the most typical cases of obsession the sufferer has an unpleasant intrusive thought which he often recognizes to be irrational but which he is not able to dismiss. Typical thoughts are that he will hurt or kill someone. ... The intrusive thoughts, however, are accompanied by further unreasonable thoughts to the effect that the sufferer will be responsible for harm and will be blamed. The behaviour which is compulsive – endless washing, hiding away potential weapons etc. – is designed to neutralize the risk of harm and blame'. (Observe that Melville (1991) treats obsessions and phobias (see below) together, thereby emphasizing their similarities.)

The authors mention a variety of obsessive acts, comprising checking proce-dures, extreme cleanliness, and other rituals. A person may feel that he or she has to check the taps in the bathroom a great number of times, and the person does so although he or she clearly remembers that the tap has been checked before. The latter is an important criterion when it comes to distinguishing the case of obsession from the case of a genuine memory problem. According to Leff and Isaacs, a further criterion is that the subject performs the checks with some resistance. A conflict of wants should be clearly felt for the diagnosis of obsession to apply. The acts actually performed should, moreover, be judged by the subject as silly or, indeed, irrational.

Leff and Isaacs (1990) also make the following general comment, which has relevance for my definition of health. 'Many normal people check once or twice that they have turned off gas taps, switches and water taps, and that they have closed windows and locked doors. It is only when these procedures become time-consuming or interfere with other activities that they should be consid-ered pathological' (p. 88). The obsessional acts are considered *pathological* only when they interfere with other acts – presumably such acts as are consid-ered important by the subject. It is not the abnormality of the behaviour as such that is pathological.

The general theory of health that is suggested, although not developed, by Leff and Isaacs seems, therefore, to be in line with the holistic theories of health. What is lacking in the statement quoted is the emphasis on the *inability* of the subject to do otherwise than he or she does. On the other hand, this feature is quite clear in other parts of the characterization of the obsessive condition.

With obsessional acts, a salient case of a conflict of wants exists, where the most irrational want happens to be the one which is acted upon. The question now is how this case should be classified according to my basic analysis and taxonomy. Having a conflict of wants is not in itself either irrational or patho-logical. The irrationality may be contained in the fact that the act chosen stems from an *irrational* want. What species of irrational want is this in its turn? It is too much to say that it is of a self-destructive kind. The whole pattern of obsessional acting may ultimately become self-destructive, but the single act of checking one's bathroom taps ten times is not self-destructive. I think that we must say that the irrationality here is ultimately one of beliefs. The subject believes, at least at certain moments, that a risk exists that the water is still running from the tap. At other moments, or indeed at the same time, he or she believes that this cannot possibly be so. Subjectively, overwhelming evidence also exists that the taps have been turned off. The situation can perhaps be described as follows: the subject cannot help having a completely unjustified, indeed foolish, belief. This, however, is hardly the whole analysis. The compelling unjustified belief would not issue in a want to check the taps unless the agent wanted quite strongly to avoid having a running tap. A running tap is normally not seen as a disastrous state of affairs. The person with the obsession, however, must have made a very strong negative evaluation of it.

The condition of obsessional acts could then, in my terms, be analysed as, first, a case of incoherence of beliefs or, more precisely, of the possession of a subjectively unjustified set of beliefs that the subject cannot avoid having, although he or she sincerely wants to avoid having them, and second, a strong want to avoid the risk that a certain state of affairs presents. It is not customary, however, to classify the beliefs held in obsessions as delusions. The reason for this reluctance is perhaps that the beliefs in obsessions, although foolish, are not considered to be blatantly absurd.

I have used the term 'compelling' in discussing the condition of obsession. First, the textbook authors use it. I also use the term 'compelling unjustified belief'. The question is now if obsession fulfils the criteria of being a compelling condition in the technical sense characterized above. Two points have to be made here. First, in my analysis, it is primarily *the belief* that the tap is running that is compelling. The subject cannot avoid having this belief. But, second, also an intention always operates in the obsessive case, namely the intention to avoid a running tap (which may be derived from various higher-order intentions, such as an intention to prevent the flat from being flooded or an intention to reduce the water bill). I have so far said that this intention must be 'strong' since the agent keeps acting on it many times. Also, the agent may not be prepared to relinquish it under any circumstances whatsoever. If this is the case, then the obsessive action also fulfils the condition of being a compelled act in my technical sense.

Both similarities and dissimilarities exist between the beliefs that lie behind obsessional acts and what are called *obsessional thoughts* in psychiatric literature. Consider the characterization in Leff and Isaacs (1990): 'There are unpleasant thoughts, often with a violent, sexual, or distasteful content, which repeatedly force themselves into the patient's mind against his will. They are repetitive in nature and are repellent or even horrifying to the patient, who resists them strongly but unsuccessfully' (p. 90). The authors underline that the thoughts that force themselves upon the patients should not be confused with the subcase of delusional thought insertion. The patients with delusional thought insertion believe that their thoughts arise from the outside. This never occurs with obsessional thoughts.

Leff and Isaacs, and this is certainly in accordance with psychiatric praxis, delimit here a class that is both narrower and wider than a set of beliefs that the subject cannot avoid having. The class is narrower in the sense that the obsessional thoughts, according to the definition, should in themselves be extremely unpleasant to the subject. The belief that a tap is running, however, is hardly in itself very unpleasant. The class delimited is wider in the sense that the obsessional thoughts need not be of a belief kind; they could be thoughts depicting a merely possible state of affairs not believed by the subject to be realized.

9.3.4 **Phobic anxiety**

Marks (1969, p.3) defines a phobia as a special form of fear that (1) is out of proportion to the demands of the situation, (2) cannot be explained or resolved away, (3) is beyond voluntary control, and (4) leads to avoidance of the feared situation. Leff and Isaacs (1990, p.86) add: 'For this symptom to be judged present, the patient should complain of anxiety which is linked with particular objects or situations. ... The situations which commonly engender phobic anxiety are open spaces, enclosed spaces, travelling in a vehicle, being left alone, being in crowds, and meeting people'. Charlton (1988, p. 158) provides the following characterization: 'A *phobia* is an aversion to something the agent thinks good. *Malakia* (a milder variant) is aversion to doing what you think you should do because it is unpleasant'.

I have in practice already made an analysis of this case. The analysis can be performed in three steps. On the first level, the problem consists either in the fact (a) that a person cannot achieve certain specific objectives, for instance walk to his or her workplace, because this would involve travelling in vehicles and being in crowds – and the person cannot do this because it creates an intolerable degree of anxiety – or in the general fact (b) that the person so often feels such anxiety (since moving around among people is almost unavoidable) that his or her general ability to cope with life is grossly impaired. On the second level, we can make the abstract observation that the phobia consists in a conflict between a set of basic wants that the person has and a strong fear. According to the analysis of emotions that I have presented above, this conflict is basically tantamount to a conflict between wants, for instance the basic want to go to one's work and the want to avoid the tremendous danger of being in a crowd. The latter want – and now we are coming to the third level of analysis – is dependent on a belief that is unjustified. The subject must believe (at least at times) that a crowd is intrinsically highly dangerous. Since a lot of evidence to the contrary exists, the subject also appears to be incapable of avoiding this belief.

The analysis of phobic anxiety, as long as we perform this analysis exclusively along dimensions of rationality, parallells the analysis of obsession very closely. (Marks (1969, pp. 139–140) also explicitly connects phobias with obsessions in his analysis.) My characterization is of course far from exhaustive as a description of the phenomena in their entirety. A salient difference between the two exists insofar as the phobia entails a strong *feeling* of anxiety; I am here referring to the sensational element of an emotion that is left out in a pure want-belief analysis of emotions.

9.3.5 The rigid personality

Löw-Beer (2004) makes an interesting analysis of the rigid personality type, which has a clear affinity to my analysis of compulsion in the psychiatric context. Löw-Beer argues that rigidity is 'wrong because it is irrational and objectively compulsive' (p. 258). The rigid person has no choice. He or she has no alternative to the rigid way of life. On the other hand, the rigid person does not necessarily feel forced to do what he or she does. (I am not here presupposing that a rigid person is a mentally disturbed person in the *DSM* sense; nor does Löw-Beer in his article. It seems clear, however, that rigidity is a central element in the minds of certain mentally disturbed persons.)

Löw-Beer does not attempt to give a strict definition of rigidity. However, he provides a sufficiently rich description of the typically rigid person for us to judge what such a person has in common with the mentally disturbed persons discussed in this chapter. Rigidity for Löw-Beer is a character trait that entails quite a narrow life lacking alternative courses of action. The rigid person often has a very strong sense of duty and feels obliged to comply with the duties. What distinguishes the rigid person from an ordinary dutiful person is that the rigid person has in a sense invented or created many of the duties him- or herself. The rigid person is the author of the duties, without normally being aware of this fact.

But why does the rigid person invent the duties? Does that not complicate life for him or her? It may do so in the end but, in the short run, it may help the person in decision making. If there is a duty for A to do F, and A is aware of this duty, then A immediately knows what should be done. The hypothesis then is that the rigid person fears making decisions. It may be the case, according to Löw-Beer's analysis, that the rigid person fears his or her own wants or fears the consequences of realizing them. Another alternative is that the rigid person has no real access to his or her wants. In order to help the decision making, the rigid person, therefore, needs external help. Clear obligations or clear rules might help. Therefore, in the absence of salient official duties or rules, the rigid person has a tendency to 'invent' the duties and rules.

In sum, the rigid person is tormented by situations of choice. He, therefore, invents 'all kinds of devices that narrow his freedom of choice' (Löw-Beer 2004, p. 265).

Löw-Beer provides a number of illustrative examples, most of them taken from Shapiro (1981). One of the mechanisms by which the rigid person arrives at 'creating' duties is to start with weak normative expectations and then turn these into strict duties. 'Thus such people feel that propriety requires them to dress neatly, duty obliges them to visit Aunt Tilly, ... mental health necessitates a number of hobbies and a certain degree of "relaxation"' (Löw-Beer 2004, p. 262 and Shapiro 1981, p. 39).

In general, Löw-Beer and Shapiro claim that the rigid person feels well as long as he or she knows what to do. When at work, the person thinks 'I am a worker', and this gives a necessary security. When at home, he or she thinks 'I am the spouse who comes in and works with my beloved family' (Löw-Beer 2004, p. 263).

How does this case relate to our analysis of compulsion in the psychiatric context? The answer, according to the analysis of Löw-Beer, could be the following. The rigid person has a fixated want to fulfil his or her duties. Thus, when the duty summons, the rigid person is compelled to comply with it. Moreover, this compliance with duties totally dominates the life of the rigid person. When official duties (or salient moral duties) are lacking, the rigid person finds and invents such duties. The subject is unaware of this process, and it would be disastrous to the whole project for him or her to become aware of it. Hence, the rigid person is in no position to withdraw the duty and eliminate the necessity. Thus, there is a case of total compulsion.

9.3.6 Psychopathy

Let me finally turn to one of the most difficult diagnoses among mental disorders and see if it can at all fit the pattern of irrational compulsion that I have sketched above. This is what is commonly called psychopathy or, formally, antisocial personality disorder (*DSM IV*). Significant features of this disorder are: failure to conform to social norms; a pattern of impulsiveness, whereby decisions are made on the spur of the moment; performance of aggressive acts; and a reckless disregard for the safety of oneself and others.

It may seem that psychopathy is quite different from the disorders cited above. Whereas the other disorders (with the possible exception of rigidity) only concern a limited part of the subject's personality, psychopathy is a condition that pervades the whole personality. A person as a whole is a psychopath. His or her complete life is (or could be) determined by this trait. But does this entail that the acts of the psychopath are entirely of a different order than the acts considered earlier in this chapter?

Let me first refer to some elements of the psychiatric discussion of psychopathy, taking Gillett (1999) as my primary guide. Gillett reminds us that what is now called psychopathy was for a long time known as a kind of *moral* insanity. The insanity of the psychopaths is to a great extent expressed in immoral, even criminal acts, often involving great cruelty. Many of the condemned criminals who inhabit our prisons would, according to Gillett, be labelled as psychopaths. The impression of immorality is enlarged by the fact that the psychopath is typically a highly intelligent person who is, intellectually, quite aware of the nature of the acts performed.

The question whether psychopathy could reasonably be treated as a singular disorder, where there is a kernel feature common to all instances, is highly controversial. Blackburn and Lee-Evans (1985), who did a lot of work to trace identifiable subgroups of psychopathy, ended up in scepticism in this regard. At one time, Blackburn (1988) held the opinion that ascribing psychopathy to a person is the same as giving a moral judgment masquerading as a clinical diagnosis. In any event, Blackburn settled on the view that there are at least two significant groups of people normally referred to as psychopaths.

> One group is in general terms socially outgoing, relatively free from tendencies to feel anxious or depressed. ... This group seems to represent the primary psychopath. The other, characterized by high levels of social withdrawal and emotional disturbance, appears to correspond to the category of secondary or neurotic psychopath. (Blackburn and Lee-Evans, p. 93)

The psychopathy of the second group is by and large an effect of environmental causes. These individuals tend to have a poor social and educational background, and they have an overwhelming sense that life is a series of no-win situations. They have had little social training and have never learnt successful strategies. The members of the first group can come from all social classes, are often intelligent, charming, and well-educated. Their inability must, therefore, according to Blackburn and Lee-Evans, be explained more in constitutional, biological, terms.

Gillett (1999) is more optimistic than his colleagues with regard to the characterization of psychopathy and considers that a detailed philosophical and discursive account may succeed in identifying the common phenomenology of the disorder of psychopathy. Gillett holds the view that psychopathy is a disorder of volition 'because the principal defect concerns the self-control evident in the actions of the individual towards others'. (p.263)

> The individual seems to lack any significant ability to bring his life into line with values he quite openly discusses, avows, and defends. (p.263)

Gillett thus argues along my general lines with regard to mental illness in general and psychopathy in particular. Psychopathy is a mental inability (thus an illness). Moreover, psychopathy has to do with a lack of self-control. The individual cannot control his or her impulses to perform sometimes horrendous actions. This inability to control is, in its turn, according to Gillett, due either to an inability to respond to important social cues, such as other people's reactions, or to an inability to internalize these cues into emotive or moral incitements.

A distinguished philosopher (Mackie 1977) attempts to draw an interesting and crucial line between psychopathy and other mental illnesses. Mackie discusses various reasons for excuses with regard to criminal acts, and emphasizes that the psychopaths are different from most other people who can, for psychiatric reasons, be excused for their undesired actions. Mackie thinks that people who act under duress, as well as the compulsive drinkers and the kleptomaniacs, can be excused, in line with my reasoning, because at a particular time they 'cannot do otherwise'. Moreover, Mackie says, their criminal or immoral actions are not in line with their normal personality. For Mackie, the deviance from the person's standard personality is a main criterion for excuse. The situation is quite different with the psychopath. If his or her condition is chronic, which is usually the case, then the psychopath exhibits irresponsible behaviour almost all the time. And, Mackie maintains, there is nothing compulsive about the psychopath. This person is free to act as he or she pleases.

I agree with Mackie that there are crucial differences between psychopaths and some other kinds of subjects with mental disorders. (However, psychopaths are not the only ones who can have chronic disorders.) I do not, however, agree with Mackie in his denial that the theory of compulsion is applicable to psychopaths. (It should be emphasized here that Mackie does not work with a particular theory of compulsion and that he probably has a more narrow notion of compulsion in mind.) Observe how Mackie himself describes the category of psychopaths: 'The psychopath is in some ways like a young child. Of him in particular it is plausible to say that he is not a moral agent' (p. 184). And later he goes on to say: 'Of the psychopath, then, it is correct to say that he is not responsible because he lacks the normal capacities for doing what the law requires' (p. 187).

Here, I agree entirely with Mackie. The psychopath can be considered to be ill because he or she lacks the ability to realize certain vital goals. I wish, however, to go further and say that the psychopath lacks this capacity since he or she, like the small child, is unable to weigh alternative actions and consider which action among the alternatives is the most appropriate one to perform. Thus, the psychopath is in this respect akin to the unimaginative person who cannot see that there is something else to be done. Of course, the psychopath, who is often quite intelligent, can normally in a technical sense see alternative actions, but he or she is unable to understand that some of these alternatives are to be preferred, that they ought to be performed (for instance, from a moral point of view), instead of the action in fact chosen. Thus, subjectively, given the psychopath's desires, there is, in a particular situation, only one course of action – namely the most desire-fulfilling one – available to him or her. Thus, the actions of the psychopath fulfil my criteria for compulsion.

9.4 **Summary**

Let me now summarize my theses with regard to compelled actions and mental disorders. It is my contention that many mentally disordered persons have a life-situation that is very narrow in the sense that many of their actions are compelled. The subjects have to perform (or feel that they have to perform) a particular action that is, for many reasons, undesired. They are unable to see that there is a preferable action to choose in order to reach an intended goal. The reasons for not seeing such an alternative can, however, differ. In the case of delusions (which is a common case, covering, for instance, paranoia, phobia, and possibly certain obsessions), the subjects have a set of fixated beliefs, implanted into them, which, together with their vital intentions to survive or survive unhurt, compel them to choose a particular course of action. In the case of kleptomania, pyromania, and desires brought about by alcoholism and drug addiction, it is not the belief but the want that has been inserted and fixated by a force other than the agent's self. The beliefs of these people may be completely adequate and in accordance with clear perceptions. The kleptoma- niac clearly perceives the desirable objects in the store. The pyromaniac clearly perceives a fire and, similarly, the drug addict may correctly perceive the oppor- tunity to get hold of new drugs. The rigid person implants in him- or herself a set of duties to be performed but, although the person invents these duties, this process is not accessible to him or her. Mentally retarded people, people exhibiting automatic behaviour, and psychopaths, finally, need not have any intentions or beliefs implanted in them. They are, however, for other reasons, unable to see any actions alternative to the ones they happen to choose.

It is crucial to keep in mind the general sense of compulsion that I have used throughout this study: A was compelled to do F if, and only if, A could not avoid doing F. The reason for the unavoidability need not be a strong 'force' that, in a sense, 'drags' the subject to perform a particular action. Compulsion in my sense is also the case where the agent simply does not see any alternative to a particular course of action. If there is no alternative to F-ing, and something must be done, then it is unavoidable that A does F.

Chapter 10

Epilogue

This concludes my journey from the concepts of intention and intentional action to specific forms of mental disorder. During this journey, I have attempted, in the first place, to provide a toolbox of action-theoretic concepts for the purpose of understanding what a rational action is and how such an action comes about.

The toolbox has a variety of elements. Many of these are conceptual distinctions of different kinds and orders. First, I have made the fundamental distinctions between action-types and action-instances, and between action-types of various degrees of specification. Second, I have noted that actions may be distinguished along dimensions of complication. I have focused on two such dimensions. One dimension concerns the number of conditions in the external world that have to be fulfilled in order for an action of a certain type to occur. This led me to the fundamental distinction between natural actions and conventional actions, the latter being actions that have come into being through conventional stipulation. The second dimension concerns how actions can be added to each other to form action-complexes, these I have called action-chains and action-sequences. Furthermore, I have distinguished between intentional, voluntary, and compelled actions, and between rational and irrational actions. All this has laid the ground for an explication of the notions of rational explanation and rational determination.

Connected to this general treatment of action and rational action, I have presented an analysis of the notion of ability. Ability and its various species can easily be traced once we understand the variety of actions, from basic actions to the most complex generated actions in the form of action-chains and action-sequences. Ability is, in its turn, the most central concept in my theory of health and illness. Health is in my understanding to be described as a person's second-order ability to realize his or her vital goals given standard or reasonable circumstances. In a special chapter, I have applied this understanding of health to the mental arena and analysed the notion of a mental ability and, subsequently, mental health.

These parallel investigations have brought me to the topic of mental disorder. I have first tested the traditional idea that irrationality should be the kernel element in mental disorder. I have distinguished several types of irrationality, from false beliefs to incomplete practical syllogisms, and tried to see what role they may play as essential features of mental disorder. My preliminary conclusion is that irrationality as such is never a sufficient criterion of mental disorder. I have two principal arguments for this conclusion. First, irrationality in various forms and degrees is an ingredient in every human being's life. What is significant for most people is, however, that they can control and correct most variants of their irrationality, if they choose to. They can correct their unfounded beliefs, and they can improve on their reasoning. Most people are free to make such a choice. A person with a mental disorder is typically not free to do so. Second, following my own analysis of the notions of health and illness, irrationality should be regarded as pathological only if it prevents the subject from realizing any of his or her vital goals. Such irrationality that is no trouble to the subject does not cause or constitute illness. In this regard, I am close to the view expressed in the definition of mental disorder in *DSM IV*.

In some previous studies (1995; 2001) (summarized in this volume), I have attempted to give characterizations of the general notions of health and illness. My treatise in this book does not have such a general ambition with regard to mental disorder (as opposed to physical illness). However, during the journey, I have indicated some possible routes towards a definition of mental disorder without developing these in any detail (see Chapter 3, Section 3.2). Instead, I have concentrated on an explication of some crucial mental disorders centring around the phenomena of delusion and irresistible desires. Here, the action-theoretic toolbox can be put to maximal use.

Previous studies have suggested that many mental disorders in this area involve actions that the subject is in some sense not free to choose or avoid. Typically, the subject is, or feels that he or she is, compelled to act in a certain way. This element of compulsion is essential. It is the compulsion that makes the condition detrimental and forces the subject to perform actions that prevent the realization of his or her vital goals.

Hence, my focus has gradually moved towards an explication of the concept of compulsion. I have made this analysis partially in dispute with certain specialists in the field, such as Wertheimer and Audi. My general idea is that the notion of compulsion that is relevant in psychiatry is one tied to subjective unavoidability. This notion, in its turn, is based on the idea of fixation of intentions and convictions (beliefs or other experiences). A person A is subjectively compelled to perform a certain action F if, and only if, A's intentions and convictions are fixated in the sense that A cannot, or is absolutely not prepared to, change them. The fixation may be due to the subject's own choice, but, in the case of mental disorder, it is typical that at least one of the two types (intention or conviction) has been implanted without the agent's own making. In special cases of mental disorder, such as automatism, the fixation may be due to the unavailability of alternative intentions and/or convictions. Finally, I have attempted to exemplify this phenomenon from psychiatric literature. I have found that my analysis can be applied, for instance, to the phenomena of paranoia, pathological drives such as kleptomania and pyromania, obsessions, phobia, rigidity, and psychopathy.

If there is anything useful in this intellectual journey, it may be seen as one where insights from one discipline – philosophical action theory – can be used to clarify concepts in certain other disciplines, such as abnormal psychology and psychiatry.

Part 3

Summary of Basic Concepts

Glossary

In the following, I list and explain the most crucial concepts used in this book. Only a few of these concepts have been defined in a strict way. Others have been more informally described, whereas yet others have only been commented on. The presentation below mirrors the level of specification given in the book.

Action-theoretic notions

Action An episode involving both an agent A and the result brought about by the agent. A performs an action F if, and only if, A intentionally makes F the case.

Basic action A basic action is an action that does not presuppose the performance of any other action by the agent A. A basic action typically involves only a bodily movement: for instance, A moves his finger.

Generated action A generated action presupposes the performance of at least one other action. One of these must be a basic action. Example: A fired his gun by moving his finger. The mechanism by which the generation is performed can be either causal, as in this example, or conventional. An example of the latter type is: B opened her bank account by signing her name.

Action chain An action chain is defined by a basic action and all its generated actions.

Action sequence An action sequence is constituted by a series of basic actions (and their action chains) held together by a common intention.

Intention An intention is a mental state of a person, namely a variant of the person's will. An intention may or may not be the result of a decision. An intention is a kind of strong will. An intention to perform the action F is always acted upon if it lasts to the time when it is supposed to issue in action. This means that B will attempt to perform F at t if B intends to perform F at t. B may, however, fail to realize F, if she lacks the capacity or if she is prevented by external phenomena.

Want A want is a type of will that is weaker than an intention. A may want to do F at t without attempting to do F at t even if A does not lack the capacity for doing F nor is impeded by an external obstacle. A reason for this may be a conflicting want. A want may be defined as a disposition to form an intention.

Emotion An emotion is a mental state of the feeling type. Emotions differ from other types of feeling, for instance sensations and moods, by being directed towards objects. Example: A fears the wolf, or A is in love with a woman. Most emotions are conceptually connected to a certain situational fact, which is called the reason for the emotion. Example: John was afraid because a dangerous animal approached him.

Intentional explanation of actions In this book, I normally refer to a complete explanatory schema of the following type, also called a *PSI* (practical syllogism involving an intention):

A intends to bring about P

A believes that he is in situation C

A believes that he will not bring about P in C unless he does F

A can do F in C

A sets himself to do F

Reason for action In this book, reason has one narrower and one wider use. In the more narrow use, a reason is a fact (normally a fact external to the agent) that rationalizes and explains an action. Example: The fact that it was raining prompted A to fetch an umbrella. A reason, thus, takes the position of C in the intentional explanation of actions. In a wider sense, other explanatory factors also can be called reasons. An exception, though, is the intention itself. A reason is always a reason in the light of an intention (or a want, see below).

Practical syllogism of wants (PSW) A situation of deliberation can be described by a schema that is structurally similar to the intentional explanatory one *(PSI)*.

A wants to bring about P

A believes that he is in situation C

A believes that he will not bring about P in C unless he does F

A believes that he can do F

If A does not have a conflicting want, then the *PSW* typically leads to a decision to do F. If, moreover, the capacity clause if fulfilled, the *PSW* turns into a *PSI*.

Understanding an action To understand an action is (in this book) to correctly identify the action. A correct identification entails getting hold of the intention with which the agent acted.

Ability Ability and opportunity are complementary concepts in the sense that if B has the ability and opportunity to do F, then B has the practical possibility to do F. The word 'can' that is used in the practical syllogisms above signifies practical possibility. If it is practically possible for B to do F, it means that B succeeds in performing F if she tries to perform F.

A person's ability is based on her internal physical and mental conditions. This person's opportunity for the same action is constituted by the external physical or conventional conditions.

In this book, ability normally refers to the ability to perform intentional actions. For a discussion of a deviant case, see Chapter 3, Section 3.2.

Second-order ability Ability as described above can also be called first-order ability. It can be distinguished from second-order ability, which can be given the following definition: A has a second-order ability with regard to an action F if, and only if, A has the first-order ability to pursue a training programme after the completion of which A will have the first-order ability to do F.

Opportunity See ability.

Practical possibility See ability.

Competence A person's competence with regard to an action F is a part of the person's full ability to perform F. It is typical that competence is an enduring state of a person that is the result of education and training. Competence is, however, compatible with lack of full ability. The competent person may, for temporal reasons (such as ill health), have lost his or her executive ability to perform F.

Mental action A mental action is one that issues from one of the mental faculties, namely the cognitive, emotional, or conative faculties, and does not involve any bodily movements.

Mental ability By mental ability, I refer both to a person's ability to perform an intentional mental action and to a person's disposition to enter a particular mental state. Example of the latter: A has the ability to fall in love or B lacks the ability to feel remorse.

Compulsion The general sense of compulsion as understood in this book is the following: A was compelled to do F at t if, and only if, A could not avoid doing F at t in the light of A's intentions and beliefs at t. The reason why A could not avoid doing F is typically that A's intentions and beliefs were fixated, which means either that they could not be altered by A himself or that A was not prepared to alter them.

Coercion. Coercion is that species of compulsion where a human being intentionally compels another agent to perform a certain action.

Cognitive notions

Cognition This term is here used as an umbrella term for a number of epistemic concepts, primarily beliefs, convictions, understandings, and acts of knowing. Common to all cognitions is that they are mental states that in one way or the other entertain the reality of a fact.

Irrational belief This book analyses a number of senses of irrational beliefs. Two examples follow.

    Incoherent belief *A* has an incoherent belief if, and only if, *A* believes in a contradiction, such as *p* and *non-p*.

    Unjustified belief A belief is unjustified if it is not supported by any empirical or logical evidence. A distinction is made between objectively justified and subjectively justified beliefs.

Irrational want This book analyses a number of senses of irrational wants. Three examples follow.

    Illogical want-structure *A* has an illogical want structure if, and only if, *A* wants to have *P*, is convinced that *Q* is necessary for *P*, and does not have any reason for rejecting either *P* or *Q*, but still does not want *Q*.

    Unrealistic want A want can be both objectively and subjectively unrealistic. The latter case concerns a person who wants to achieve something but is convinced that he or she cannot achieve it.

    Self-destructive want The ultimately self-destructive want is one that cannot be rationalized by any other want, such as wanting to defend a person or realizing a higher goal.

Health-theoretic notions

Health In this book I have proposed the following formal definition of health: *A* is completely healthy if, and only if, *A* is in a bodily and mental state such that *A* has the second-order ability to realize all his or her vital goals, given a set of standard or otherwise reasonable circumstances.

Vital goal A vital goal of *A*'s is a state of affairs that is necessary for this person's long-term minimal happiness.

Standard circumstance A standard circumstance is a state of affairs (physical or conventional) that is assumed to be standard in a particular society.

Disease A disease is such a bodily or mental state in a person that tends to make him ill. The person is ill if his or her state of health has been substantially reduced.

Mental illness A person is mentally ill if, and only if, this person's health has been substantially reduced by mental causes, such as depression, anxiety or delusions.

Psychiatric notions

Mental disorder (the sense of *DSM IV*). This book frequently refers to the definition of mental disorder proposed in the *Diagnostic Manual of Mental Disorders (IV)*. It runs as follows: 'Each of the mental disorders is conceptualised as a clinically significant behavioural or psychological syndrome or pattern that occurs in an individual and that is associated with present distress (e.g. a painful symptom) or disability (i.e. an impairment in one or more important areas of functioning) or with a significantly increased risk of suffering, death, pain, disability, or an important loss of freedom' (1994, p. XII).

Akrasia or weak will is the case 'when a person is irrational by his own lights; he recognises what he ought to do, but fails to do it' (Hurley 1989).

Delusion Delusion is a central psychiatric concept that has been given several definitions, some of which are discussed in this book (Chapter 9, Section 9.1). The definition given in *DSM IV* is the following: 'A false belief based upon incorrect inference about external reality that is firmly sustained despite what almost everyone else believes and despite what constitutes incontrovertible and obvious proof or evidence to the contrary. The belief is not one ordinarily accepted by other members of the person's culture or subculture (e.g. it is not an article of religious faith)' (1994, p. 765).

Paranoia Paranoia (or delusional disorder) is conceived of as a disorder of various types, for instance erotomanic, grandiose, jealous, and persecutory type. In this book, the persecutory type is focused on. 'This subtype applies when the central theme of the delusion involves the person's belief that he or she is being conspired against, cheated, spied on, followed, poisoned or drugged, maliciously maligned, harassed or obstructed in the pursuit of long-term goals' (*DSM IV*, p. 298).

Automatism Automatism 'means unconscious, involuntary action ... [it could be explained] simply as action without any knowledge of acting, or action with no consciousness of doing what was being done' (Reznek 1997, p. 93).

Kleptomania 'Kleptomania is the recurrent failure to resist impulses to steal items even though the items are not needed for personal use or for their monetary value' (*DSM IV*, p. 612.)

Pyromania Pyromania entails 'the presence of multiple episodes of deliberate and purposeful fire setting. Individuals with the disorder experience tension or affective arousal before setting a fire' (*DSM IV*, p. 614).

Obsession Obsessional acts are 'repetitive acts, usually commonplace in nature, which the patient feels compelled to carry out although he resists them as unnecessary or even stupid' (Leff and Isaacs 1990, p. 88).

Phobic anxiety 'For phobic anxiety to be judged present, the patient should complain of anxiety which is linked with particular objects or situations. ... The situations which commonly engender phobic anxiety are open spaces, enclosed spaces, travelling in a vehicle, being left alone, being in crowds, and meeting people' (Leff and Isaacs 1990, p. 86).

Rigid personality Rigidity is a character trait that entails a narrow life, lacking alternative courses of action. The rigid person often has a strong sense of duty and feels obliged to comply with the duties. What distinguishes the rigid person from an ordinary dutiful person is that the rigid person has, in a sense, invented or created many of the duties him- or herself. (Summary from Löw-Beer 2004)

Psychopathy Psychopathy, or anti-social personality disorder, 'is a pervasive pattern of disregard for, and violation of, the rights of others that begins in childhood or early adolescence and continues into adulthood' (*DSM IV*, p. 645). Among the diagnostic criteria of anti-social personality disorder are the following:
1. Failure to conform to social norms with respect to lawful behaviours as indicated by repeatedly performing acts that are grounds for arrest
2. Deceitfulness, as indicated by repeated lying, use of aliases, or conning others for personal profit or pleasure
3. Impulsiveness or failure to plan ahead
4. Irritability and aggressiveness, as indicated by repeated physical fights or assaults.

References

Amador X.F. and Kronengold H. (2004) The Description and Meaning of Insight in Psychosis. In X.F. Amador and A.S. David (eds.) *Insight and Psychosis*. Oxford: Oxford University Press, pp. 15–32.

Anscombe G.E.M. (1963) *Intention*. Oxford: Blackwells.

Aristotle (1908) *The Works of Aristotle. Vol. VIII Metaphysica*. Translated into English under the editorship of Sir David Ross. Oxford: Clarendon Press.

Aristotle (1934) *The Nicomachean Ethics*, The Loeb Classical Library. London: William Heinemann Ltd.

Armstrong D. (1968) *A Materialist Theory of the Mind*. London: Routledge & Kegan Paul.

Audi R. (1993) *Action, Intention, and Reason*. Ithaka: Cornell University Press.

Austin J.L. (1975) *How to Do Things with Words*. Second edition. Cambridge, Mass.: Harvard University Press.

Bennett J. (1988) *Events and Their Names*. Oxford: Oxford University Press.

Blackburn R. (1988) On Moral Judgements and Personality Disorders: The Myth of Psychopathic Personality Revisited. *British Journal of Psychiatry*, **153**, 505–512.

Blackburn R. and Lee-Evans J.M. (1985) Reactions of Primary and Secondary Psychopaths to Anger-Evoking Situations. *British Journal of Clinical Psychology*, **24**, 93–100.

Bolton D. (2003) Meaning and Causal Explanations in the Behavioural Sciences. In K.W.M. Fulford, K. Morriss, J. Sadler, and G. Stanghellini (eds.) *Nature and Narrative: An Introduction to the New Philosophy of Psychiatry*. Oxford: Oxford University Press, pp. 113–125.

Bolton D. and Hill J. (2003) *Mind, Meaning, and Mental Disorder: The Nature of Causal Explanation in Psychology and Psychiatry*. Second edition. Oxford: Oxford University Press.

Boorse C. (1977) Health as a Scientific Concept. *Philosophy of Science*, **44**, 542–573.

Boorse C. (1997) A Rebuttal on Health. In J. Humber and R. Almeder (eds.) *What is Disease?* Totowa, N.J.: Humana Press, pp. 1–134.

Buchanan A. and Wessely S. (2004) Delusions, Action, and Insight. In X.F. Amador and A.S. David (eds.) *Insight and Psychosis*. Oxford: Oxford University Press, pp. 241–268.

Canguilhem G. (1978) *On the Normal and the Pathological*. Dordrecht: D. Reidel Publishing Company.

Chapman L.J. and Chapman J.P. (1973) *Disordered Thought and Schizophrenia*. Englewood Cliffs, N.J.: Prentice Hall Inc.

Charlton W. (1988) *Weakness of Will*. Oxford: Blackwell.

Culver C. and Gert B. (1982) *Philosophy in Medicine*. Oxford: Oxford University Press.

Cutting J. (1999) *Psychopathology & Modern Philosophy*. Scaynes Hill, West Sussex: The Forest Publishing Company.

Davidson D. (1980) *Essays on Actions and Events*. Oxford: Clarendon Press.

Dray W.H. (1957) *Laws and Explanation in History*. Oxford: Oxford University Press.

DSM IV (1994) *Diagnostic and Statistical Manual of Mental Disorders*. Washington D.C.: The American Psychiatric Association.

Freud S. (1915/1957) The Unconscious. In J. Strachey (ed.) *The Standard Edition of the Complete Psychological Works of Sigmund Freud, Vol. XIV*. London: Hogarth Press, pp. 166–208.

Fried Y. and Agassi J. (1976) *Paranoia: A Study in Diagnosis*. Dordrecht: D. Reidel Publishing Company.

Fulford K.W.M. (1989) *Moral Theory and Medical Practice*. Cambridge: Cambridge University Press.

Fulford K.W.M. (2004) Insight and Delusion: From Jaspers to Kraepelin and Back Again via Austin. In X.F. Amador and A.S. David (eds.) *Insight and Psychosis: Awareness of Illness in Schizophrenia and Related Disorders*. Oxford: Oxford University Press, pp. 51–78.

Galen (1997) *Selected Works*. Translated with an introduction and notes by P.N. Singer. Oxford: Oxford University Press.

Gardner S. (1993) *Irrationality and the Philosophy of Psychoanalysis*. Cambridge: Cambridge University Press.

Gelder M., Gath D., and Mayou R. (1989) *Oxford Textbook of Psychiatry*. Second edition. Oxford: Oxford University Press.

Gillett G. (1999) *The Mind and its Discontents: An Essay in Discursive Psychiatry*. Oxford: Oxford University Press.

Gipps R.G.T. and Fulford K.W.M. (2004) Understanding the Clinical Concept of Delusion: From an Estranged to an Engaged Epistemology. *International Review of Psychiatry* (Special Issue on the Philosophy of Psychiatry), **16**, 225–235.

Glover J. (1970) *Responsibility*. London: Routledge & Kegan Paul.

Goldman A.I. (1970) *A Theory of Human Action*. Englewood Cliffs, N.J.: Prentice Hall Inc.

Heil J. and Mele A. (eds.) (1993) *Mental Causation*. Oxford: Oxford University Press.

Hempel C. (1963) Reasons and Covering Laws in Historical Explanation. In S. Hook (ed.) *Philosophy and History*. New York: New York University Press, pp. 143–163.

Hempel C. (1965) Aspects of Scientific Explanation. In C. Hempel (ed.) *Aspects of Scientific Explanation and Other Essays in the Philosophy of Science*. New York: The Free Press, pp. 331–496.

Hurley S.L. (1989) *Natural Reasons: Personality and Polity*. Oxford: Oxford University Press.

ICD (1977) *Manual of the International Classification of Diseases, Injuries and Causes of Death (ICD 9)*. Geneva: WHO.

ICF (2001) *International Classification of Functioning, Disability and Health*. Geneva: WHO.

ICIDH (1980) *International Classification of Impairments, Disabilities, and Handicaps*. Geneva: WHO.

Jaspers K. (1913/1963) *General Psychopathology*. Translated by J. Hoenig and M.W. Hamilton. Chicago: The University of Chicago Press.

Kenny A. (1963) *Action, Emotion and Will*. London: Routledge & Kegan Paul.

Kenny A. (1975) *Will, Freedom and Power*. Oxford: Blackwell.

Kihlstrom J.F. and Hoyt I.P. (1988) Hypnosis and the Psychology of Delusions. In T.F. Oltmanns and B.A. Maher (eds.) *Delusional Beliefs*. Chichester: John Wiley & Sons, pp. 66–109.

Kräupl-Taylor F. (1983) Descriptive and Developmental Phenomena. In M. Shepherd and O.L. Zangwill (eds.) *Handbook of Psychiatry, Vol. 1*. Cambridge: Cambridge University Press, pp. 59–94.

Leff J.P. and Isaacs A.D. (1990) *Psychiatric Examination in Clinical Practice*. Third edition. Oxford: Blackwell Scientific Publications.

Leontiev A.N. (1981) The Problem of Activity in Psychology. In J.W. Wertsch (ed.) *The Concept of Activity in Soviet Psychology*. Armonk, N.Y.: M.E. Sharpe, pp. 37–71.

Löw-Beer M. (2004) Rigidity: The Strange Preference for Compulsion. In T. Schramme and J. Thome (eds.) *Philosophy and Psychiatry*. Berlin: Walter de Gruyter, pp. 257–269.

Mackie J. (1974) *The Cement of the Universe*. Oxford: Oxford University Press.

Mackie J. (1977) The Grounds of Responsibility. In P.M.S. Hacker and J. Raz (eds.) *Law, Morality and Society: Essays in Honour of H.L.A. Hart*. Oxford: Clarendon Press, pp. 175–188.

Maher B.A. (1974) Delusional Thinking and Perceptual Disorder. *Journal of Individual Psychology*, **30**, 98–113.

Maher B.A. (1988a) Anomalous Experience and Delusional Thinking: The Logic of Explanations. In T.F. Oltmanns and B.A. Maher (eds.) *Delusional Beliefs*. Chichester: John Wiley & Sons, pp. 15–33.

Maher B.A. (1988b) Language Disorders in Psychoses and Their Impact on Delusions. In M. Spitzer, F.A. Uehlein, and G. Oepen (eds.) *Psychopathology and Philosophy*. Berlin: Springer-Verlag, pp. 109–120.

Marchetti C. and della Sala S. (1998) Disentangling the Alien and Anarchic Hand. *Cognitve Neuropsychiatry*, **3**, 191–207.

Marks I.M. (1969) *Fears and Phobias*. London: William Heinemann Ltd., pp. 109–120.

Matthews E. (2003) How Can a Mind be Sick? In K.W.M. Fulford, K. Morriss, J. Sadler and G. Stanghellini (eds.) *Nature and Narrative: An Introduction to the New Philosophy of Psychiatry*. Oxford: Oxford University Press, pp. 75–92.

Melden A.I. (1961) *Free Action*. Oxford: Oxford University Press.

Mele A.R. (ed.) (1997) *The Philosophy of Action*. Oxford: Oxford University Press.

Melville J. (1991) *Phobias and Obsessions*. London: MacDonald & Co.

Menninger K. (1968) *The Crime of Punishment*. New York: Viking.

Moya C.J. (1990) *The Philosophy of Action: An Introduction*. Oxford: Polity Press.

Mullen P. (1979) Phenomenology of Disordered Mental Function. In P. Hill, R. Murray, and A. Thorley (eds.) *Essentials of Postgraduate Psychiatry*. London: Academic Press, pp. 25–54.

Munro A. (1998) *Delusional Disorder*. Cambridge: Cambridge University Press.

Musalek M. (2003) Meaning and Causes of Delusions. In K.W.M. Fulford, K. Morriss, J. Sadler and G. Stanghellini (eds.) *Nature and Narrative: An Introduction to the New Philosophy of Psychiatry*. Oxford: Oxford University Press, pp. 155–169.

Neale J.M. (1988) Defensive Functions of Manic Episodes. In T.F. Oltmanns and B.A. Maher (eds.) *Delusional Beliefs*. Chichester: John Wiley & Sons, pp. 138–156.

Nordenfelt L. (1974) *Explanation of Human Actions*. Uppsala, Sweden: Philosophical Studies published by the Philosophical Society and the Department of Philosophy, University of Uppsala.

Nordenfelt L. (1992) *On Crime, Punishment and Psychiatric Care*. Stockholm: Almqvist & Wiksell International.

Nordenfelt L. (1995) *On the Nature of Health.* Second, revised edition. Dordrecht: Kluwer Academic Publishers.

Nordenfelt L. (1997) On Ability, Opportunity and Competence: An Inquiry into People's Possibility for Action. In G. Holmström-Hintikka and R. Tuomela (eds.) *Contemporary Action Theory. Vol. 1: Individual Action.* Dordrecht: Kluwer Academic Publishers, pp. 145–158.

Nordenfelt L. (2000) *Action, Ability and Health: Essays in the Theory of Action and Welfare.* Dordrecht: Kluwer Academic Publishers.

Nordenfelt L. (2001) *Health, Science, and Ordinary Language.* Amsterdam: Rodopi Publishers.

Nordenfelt L. (2003) Action Theory, Disability and ICF. *Disability and Rehabilitation,* 25, 1075–1079.

Nozick R. (1969) Coercion. In S. Morgenbesser, P. Suppes, and M. White (eds.) *Philosophy, Science, and Method.* New York: St. Martins Press, pp. 440–472.

Oltmanns T.F. (1988) Approaches to the Definition and Study of Delusions. In T.F. Oltmanns and B.A. Maher (eds.) *Delusional Beliefs.* Chichester: John Wiley, pp. 3–11.

Parsons T. (1972) Definitions of Health and Illness in the Light of American Values and Social Structure. In E.G. Jaco (ed.) *Patients, Physicians, and Illness.* New York: The Free Press, pp. 107–127.

Pears D. (1984) *Motivated Irrationality.* Oxford: Clarendon Press.

Radden J. (1985) *Madness and Reason.* London: George Allen & Unwin.

Radden J. (1996) *Divided Minds and Successive Selves: Ethical Issues in Disorders of Identity and Personality.* Cambridge, Mass.: The MIT Press.

Radden J. (2004) Identity: Personal Identity, Characterization Identity, and Mental Disorder. In J. Radden (ed.) *The Philosophy of Psychiatry: A Companion.* Oxford: Oxford University Press, pp. 133–146.

Reznek L. (1987) *The Nature of Disease.* London: Routledge & Kegan Paul.

Reznek L. (1997) *Evil or Ill?: Justifying the Insanity Defence.* London: Routledge & Kegan Paul.

Ricoeur P. (1981) *Hermenutics and the Human Sciences.* Cambridge, Mass.: Cambridge University Press.

Ryle G. (1949) *The Concept of Mind.* London: Hutchinson.

Ryle G. (1971) *Gilbert Ryle: Collected Papers, 2: Collected Essays 1929–1968.* London: Hutchinson.

Schopp R.F. (1991) *Automatism, Insanity, and the Psychology of Criminal Responsibility: A Philosophical Inquiry.* Cambridge: Cambridge University Press.

Schramme T. (2004) Coercive Threats and Offers in Psychiatry. In T. Schramme and J. Thome (eds.) *Philosophy and Psychiatry.* Berlin: Walter de Gruyter, pp. 357–369.

Searle J.R. (1969) *Speech Acts.* Cambridge: Cambridge University Press.

Searle J.R. (2001) *Rationality in Action.* Cambridge, Mass.: The MIT Press.

Shapiro D. (1981) *Autonomy and Rigidity.* New York: Basic Books.

Southard E.E. (1916) On Descriptive Analysis of Manifest Delusions from the Subject's Point of View. *Journal of Abnormal Psychology,* 11, 189–202.

Spitzer M. (1988) Karl Jaspers, Mental States, and Delusional Beliefs: A Redefinition and Its Implications. In M. Spitzer, F.A. Uehlein, and G. Oepen (eds.) *Psychopathology and Philosophy*. Berlin: Springer-Verlag, pp. 128–142.

Spitzer M., Maher B.A., and Uehlein F.A. (1990) Synopsis and Critical Remarks. In M. Spitzer and B.A. Maher (eds.) *Philosophy and Psychopathology*. Heidelberg: Springer-Verlag, pp. 223–239.

Stephens G.L. and Graham G. (2004) Reconceiving Delusions. *International Review of Psychiatry*, **16**, 236–241.

Stroud S. (2003) Weakness of Will and Practical Judgment. In S. Stroud and C. Tappolet (eds.) *Weakness of Will and Practical Irrationality*. Oxford: Oxford University Press, pp. 121–146.

Tengland P-A. (2001) *Mental Health: A Philosophical Analysis*. Dordrecht: Kluwer Academic Publishers.

Vendler Z. (1967) *Linguistics in Philosophy*. Ithaka, N.Y.: Cornell University Press.

Watson G. (1977) Skepticism About Weakness of Will. *Philosophical Review*, **86**, 316–339.

Wertheimer A. (1987) *Coercion*. Princeton, N.J.: Princeton University Press.

Westermeyer J. (1988) Some Cross-cultural Aspects of Delusions. In T.F. Oltmanns and B.A. Maher (eds.) *Delusional Beliefs*. Chichester: John Wiley and Sons, pp. 212–229.

Wittgenstein L. (1953) *Philosophical Investigations*. Oxford: Blackwells.

von Wright G.H. (1963) *Norm and Action*. London: Routledge & Kegan Paul.

von Wright G.H. (1971) *Explanation and Understanding*. London: Routledge & Kegan Paul.

von Wright G.H. (1976) Replies. In J. Manninen and R. Tuomela (eds.) *Essays on Explanation and Understanding: Studies in the Foundations of Humanities and Social Sciences*. Dordrecht: D. Reidel Publishing Company, pp. 371–413.

Index